THE EXPERT WITNESS II

THE EXPERT WITNESS

Examinations of crimes, drugs and poisons by a forensic toxicologist

A Second Dose

William J. Allender

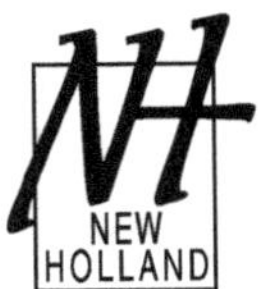

Dedication

Dedicated to the victims of the crimes and
their families, and the police officers and colleagues
I have had the privilege of working with on these,
and many other cases.

Contents

Introduction

It is a stifling-hot summer day in Sydney, Australia, with the humidity approaching the mid-nineties and a hint of an afternoon thunderstorm. A cloaked barrister blots the sweat off his brow as he strides into the courtroom, passing me in the foyer of the court waiting to give my evidence to the case at hand. One of the many participants in yet another human drama.

Hopefully, when all the evidence is presented due justice prevails, but sadly, not always ...

Poisons and drugs from a variety of sources have been used in an illegal way for centuries, and have an unfortunate, enduring fascination. People appear to be both attracted to them and at the same time repelled by them, due to the fact that they can be deadly, while they can also be very discreet. In forensic investigations, the questions that are usually raised are: Did the victim overdose? What was the poison/drug used? Was it murder, an accident or suicide? How was it taken and how much? Would that dosage be enough to take their life?

The answer will come down to how a substance was administered, probable dosage, levels found in the body, tolerance, as well as any possible motive for carrying out the deed.

As Forrest Gump said in the 1994 movie of the same name, 'Life is like a box of chocolates, you never know what you're gonna get.' And so it is with criminal cases, where some are darker than others, but none are ever sweet!

Some names in the stories presented here have been changed for legal reasons. However, I hope you the reader find these stories both interesting and informative. Some even request your assistance, if possible.

William ('Bill') J. Allender
MSc PhD, FRACI, FACBS
Forensic Medical Scientist/Toxicologist

Misty River Mystery:
The Bogle-Chandler Case

'An open marriage is nature's way of telling you
that you need a divorce.'
– Ann Landers

One of the strangest cases, I've come across in my varied career was the mysterious death of Dr Gilbert Bogle and Mrs Margaret Chandler on the banks of the Lane Cove River in Sydney on New Year's Day, 1963. Margaret Chandler, while married to her husband Geoffrey, was attracted to Gilbert 'Gib' Bogle, a senior scientist employed by the Commonwealth Scientific & Industrial Research Organisation (CSIRO) where he was carrying out research into the physics of masers, a magnetic version of lasers. It was a brief, salacious affair, which unfortunately resulted in a double tragedy.

It would be some two decades later that I would look at the case and make a curious find.

★

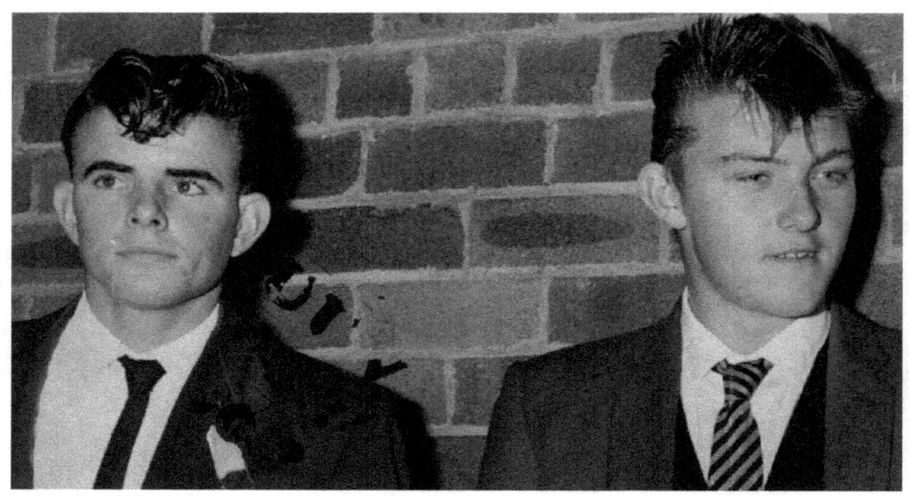

Teenagers Michael McCormick and Dennis Wheway discovered the body of Doctor Gilbert Bogle in 1963. File picture courtesy of The Daily Telegraph.

It was the morning of New Year's Day in 1963 when at 7.45 am two boys were searching the banks of the misty Lane Cove River for stray golf balls to supplement their pocket money. Unfortunately, instead of golf balls, the boys found a man in a suit lying face down on the ground on the narrow dirt track known locally as 'lovers' lane'. The boys initially thought he was just a drunk sleeping off an excess of alcohol consumed at the previous night's New Year's Eve revelries. Probably not unexpected. But when they returned to the man's body sometime later, he hadn't moved and the boys alerted police.

When Sergeant Arthur Andrews and Senior Constable Nicholls arrived in the police-issue Studebaker Lark sedan they found Bogle dead (this was further certified by a medical practitioner), but made a further bizarre discovery: he was not fully clothed as it first appeared, but was naked from the waist down. He had been covered with a piece of carpet and his suit trousers had been carefully placed over the lower part of his body. Documents on his body identified him as Dr Gilbert Stanley Bogle.

But there was more: some 18.5 metres away in a shallow depression on the edge of the river the body of a woman was found under a few sheets

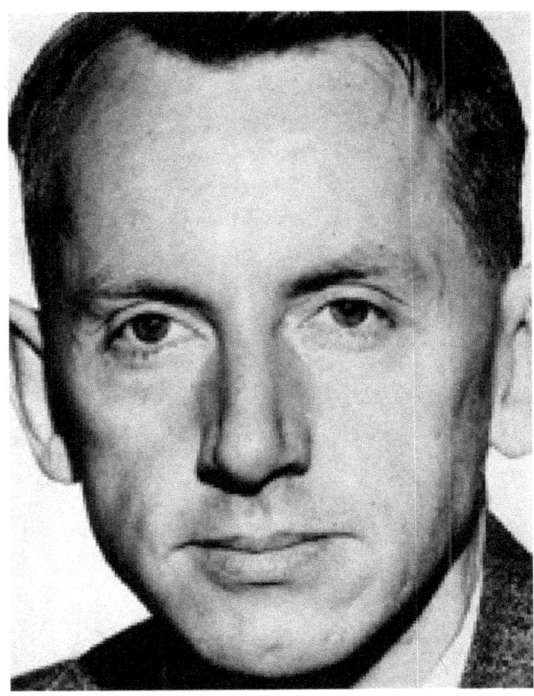

Dr Gilbert Bogle was found to have had a number of extramarital affairs. File picture courtesy of The Daily Telegraph.

of old cardboard from a broken beer box. She was lying face up and her floral frock was bunched up around her waist. In addition, her bra had been pulled down to expose her breasts. A pair of men's boxer underwear lay between her bare feet while her own panties were some metres away. The body was later identified as Mrs Margaret Olive Chandler.

While, the stench of vomit and human excreta at the crime scene made it obvious to police that the couple had been poisoned, it appeared to have taken effect while they were engaged in sexual activity, as semen was later detected on their clothing.

But, in both cases police could find no sign of violence, nor an apparent cause of death. It proved to be a very complex and difficult case with all the ingredients of an unsolved erotic murder mystery and a hint of Cold War espionage, which was to span decades.

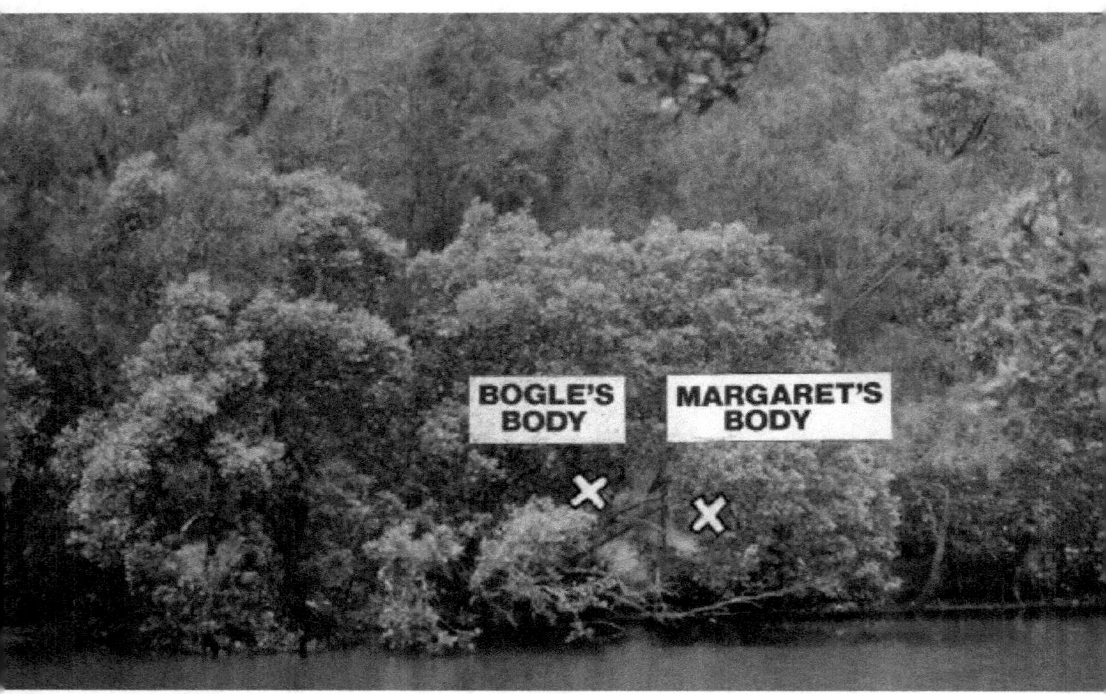

The bodies were found just metres apart.
File picture courtesy of The Daily Telegraph.

Dr Gilbert Bogle was a talented physicist and Rhodes scholar who worked at the CSIRO and was married to Vivienne Mary Bogle (Rich), a former schoolteacher and fellow graduate of Victoria University College. They had three children, one of whom was born after Gilbert's death. However, police discovered that Bogle was involved in a number of extramarital affairs with other women, many of whom he took to parks for romantic liaisons, as he had a penchant for outdoor sex.

Margaret Chandler was married to Geoffrey Arnold Chandler and the couple had two children. Mr Chandler worked as a scientific photographer in the same CSIRO building as Dr Bogle, while Mrs Chandler was a qualified nursing sister. They appear to have had an 'open marriage' and some sort of understanding that they each could

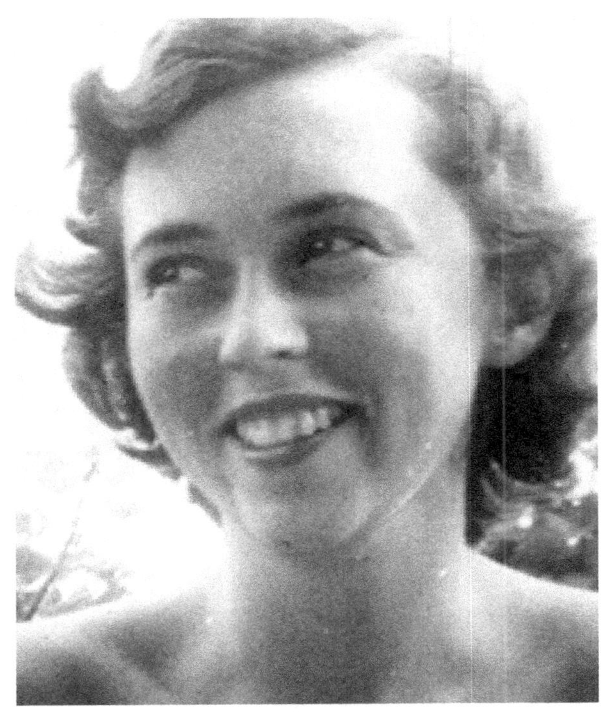

Margaret Chandler was a married mother of two.
File picture courtesy of The Daily Telegraph.

take on lovers outside their marriage. It was a strange relationship. But appeared to work for the couple.

It was just prior to Christmas 1962 that Dr Bogle, the Chandlers and a number of others, including Ken and Ruth Nash, attended a barbecue. Ken Nash also worked at the CSIRO. It was a small, relatively ordinary gathering. Dr Bogle had been the life of the party and it was soon obvious that Dr Bogle and Mrs Chandler, had 'eyes for each other'.

On the way home Mrs Chandler commented to her husband that she was quite taken with Dr Bogle. He supposedly replied, 'If you want Gib [Gilbert] as a lover, if it would you make you happy, do it.'

Geoffrey Chandler was an associate of the bohemian Sydney Push, a predominantly left-wing intellectual subculture in Sydney at the time which rejected conventional morality and authoritarianism (essentially, the lack of concern for the wishes or opinions of others). Hence, his lack of concern about his wife's interest in Gilbert Bogle. Besides, he had extramarital interests too!

Ken and Ruth Nash subsequently invited the Chandlers, along with Gilbert Bogle, to their New Year's Eve party, which was held at the Nashs' home in Waratah Street, Chatswood. Mr Chandler and his wife arrived a the party, but at about 11.30 pm Geoffrey left the party, supposedly to buy cigarettes, and drove to the suburb of Balmain where he met Pam Logan, with whom he was having an affair. He returned to the Chatswood party at about 2.30 am but left again to return to Balmain after agreeing that Dr Bogle would take Margaret Chandler home. Sometime after 4 am Dr Bogle and Mrs Chandler discreetly left the party and drove to the nearby Lane Cove River for their final sexual liaison.

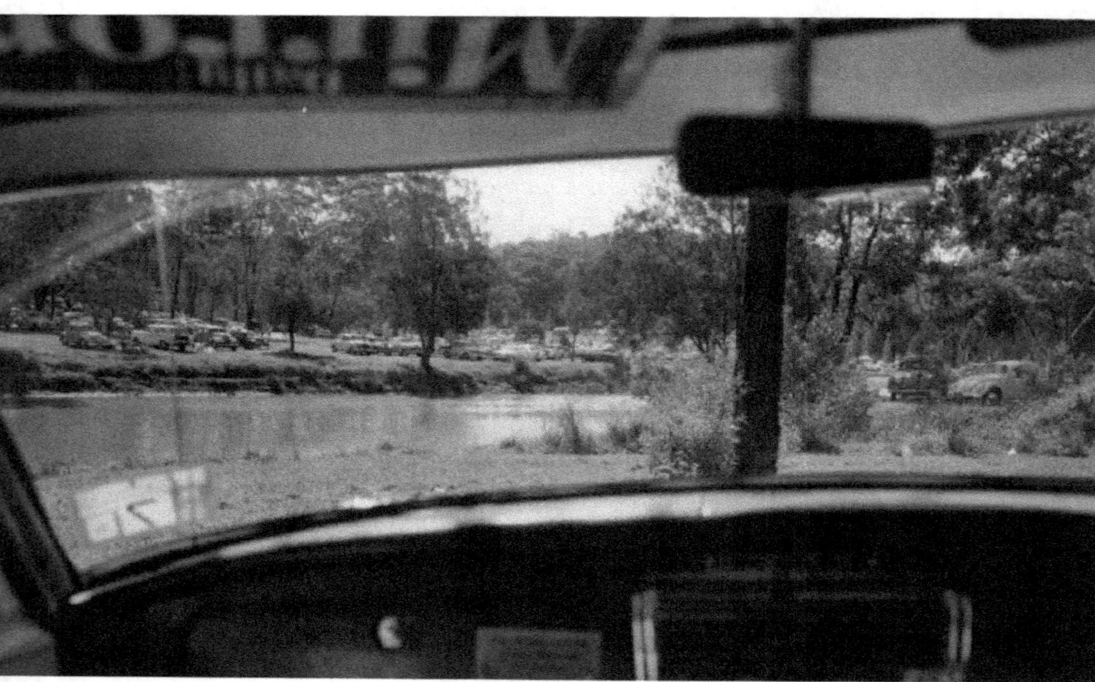

The scene from a journalist's car after it was parked in the same spot in Lane Cove National Park as Dr Bogle's car was.
File picture courtesy of The Daily Telegraph.

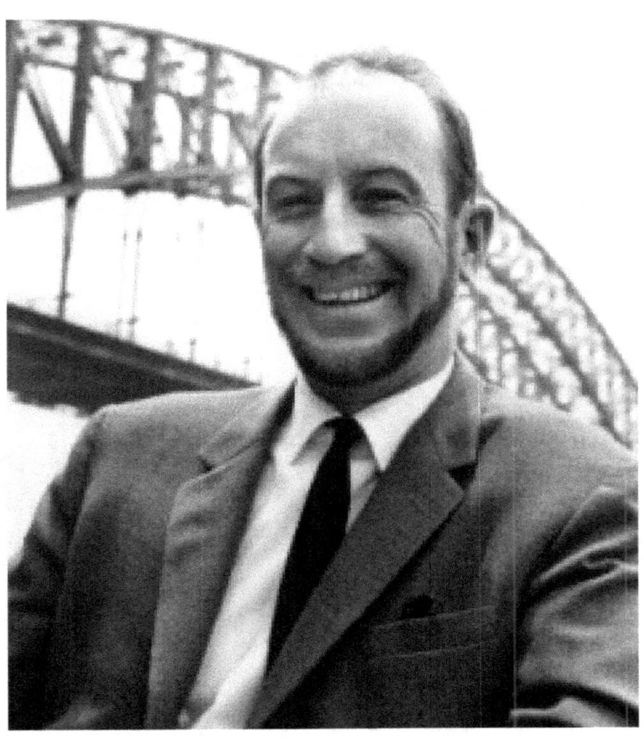

Geoffrey Chandler was Margaret's husband.
File picture courtesy of The Daily Telegraph.

It was after midday on 1 January 1963 that the Chandler and Bogle families were notified by police of the grim news of the double tragedy.

The case was soon to be widely reported, resulting in something of a media circus.

Mrs Chandler's husband Geoffrey was accused of the murders, but was never prosecuted due to lack of evidence. The most crazy (and unsupported) theory that surfaced was that Bogle was a spy, another was that the couple had taken LSD. However, none of this speculation was backed up by solid scientific evidence.

More significantly, a fellow party guest said that Bogle and Chandler appeared intoxicated at the party. Curiously, it was apparently a very staid party with a limited amount of alcohol on offer!

The autopsies on the bodies of Dr Bogle and Mrs Chandler showed no signs of violence apart from some purple/blue-coloured patches on their bodies, and the conclusion was that they had died from a poison that was never identified.

Eventually, a local greyhound trainer owned up to having found the couple early on New Year's Day morning, deciding to cover them up but also to avoid police involvement. He too was cleared of any other involvement in their deaths.

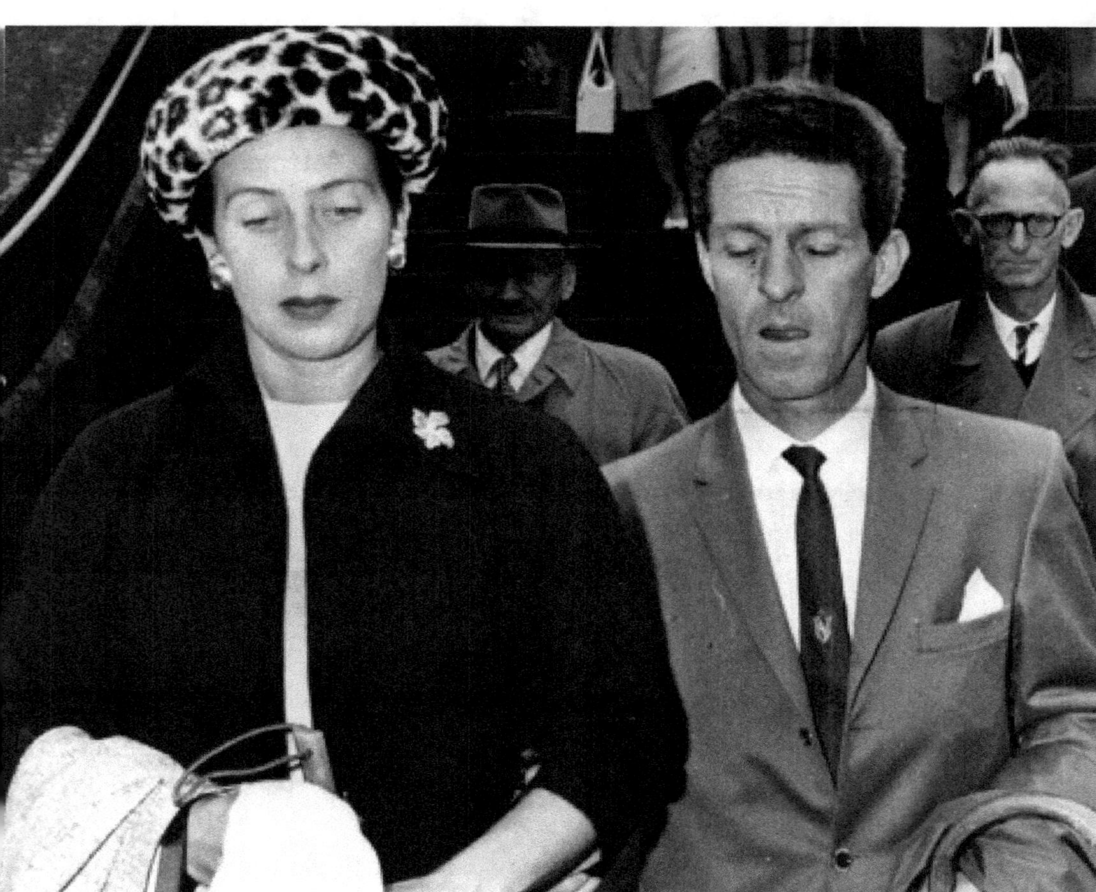

New Year's Eve party hosts Ruth and Kenneth Nash leave the inquest into the deaths. File picture courtesy of The Daily Telegraph.

At an inquest held in May 1963, the coroner, Mr J. J. Loomes, found that Dr Bogle and Mrs Chandler had died because of 'Acute circulatory failure. But as to the circumstances under which such circulatory failure was brought about, the evidence does not permit me to say.' Essentially, they died because either their hearts stopped beating or they stopped breathing.

All deaths occur because of either these failures, whether it be through ill health, poison or fatal accidents from organ damage. But, the actual cause of the deaths in this instance was unknown.

★

Fast-forward, just short of two decades after the incident, I found myself working in the Forensic Toxicology laboratory at the Division of

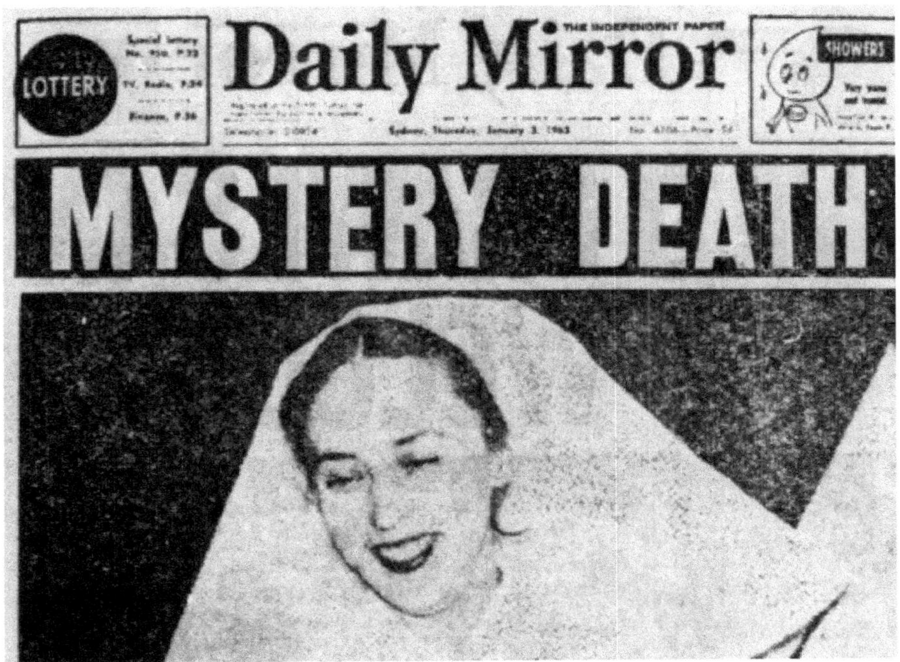

Margaret Chandler is pictured in her nurse's uniform.
File picture courtesy of The Daily Mirror.

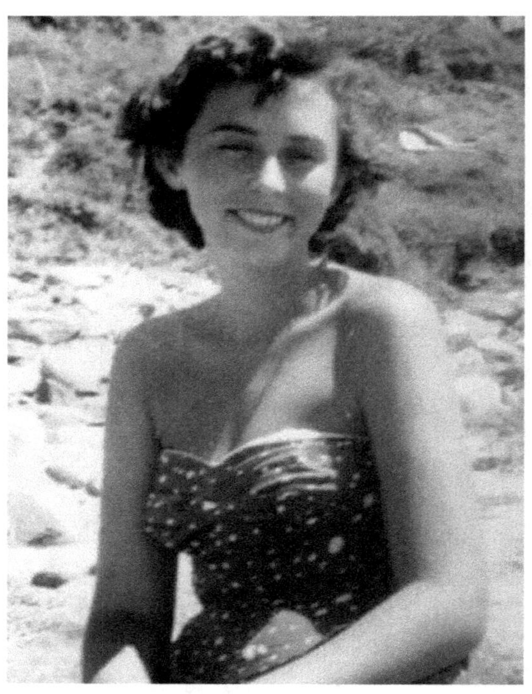

Margaret Chandler and Dr Bogle were said to have appeared intoxicated at the party they attended before their deaths.
File picture courtesy of The Daily Telegraph.

Analytical Laboratories at Lidcombe one evening in 1981, where I was employed as a forensic analyst and had to run a series of post-mortem toxicology samples on the gas chromatographs (GC) for an overnight run. The samples were extracted, but there were several other spaces left in the GC carousel. Then, I saw on entering the cool room, two samples that I thought were worth further screening. There were only two bottles of blood, one labelled 'Dr Gilbert Bogle' and the other 'Mrs Margaret Chandler'.

Unfortunately, no other organ samples were available as these had been used in earlier extensive examinations.

The blood samples were heavily haemolysed and I didn't expect much to come out of the screen. After all, some eighteen years had passed since these unfortunate, albeit controversial deaths had occurred. The

Bogle-Chandler case had become quite well-known due to the strange circumstances in which the bodies were found and also because the cause of death could not be determined. But, I thought it was still worth testing the samples, and included them in the gas chromatographic (GLC) screen. The following morning I checked the chromatograms and apart from the 'usual suspects' (caffeine etc.), the Bogle/Chandler samples were a surprise, particularly for the latter part of their chromatograms.

The earlier part of the chromatogram was a mess due to the extensively haemolysed blood. But, more importantly, there was a late eluting peak which had a Kovats index corresponding to the drug, yohimbine. It was detected in both samples – and confirmed on two chromatographic columns (OV17 and SE-30). The thin-layer chromatographic (TLC) evidence with a reference standard Rf (Retention factor) of −0.5 backed up the GLC data.

This was very unusual for two corresponding deaths.

I was now certain, based on the chromatographic evidence, that the drug responsible was yohimbine. All that was needed now was a mass spectrum of the chromatographic peaks and this would have been the clinching evidence! Unfortunately, this did not eventuate as the laboratory was in turmoil, and I was subsequently transferred to the Blood Alcohol Section.

Yohimbine is found in the barks of two evergreen trees, namely, *Pausinystalia johimbe* and *Corynanthe yohimbe* (Rubiaceae), found in parts of central and western Africa. The drug is also found in a number of other plants including *Rauwolfia Serpentina* root, also known as Indian snakeroot, or in this case, appropriately named, devil pepper. Extracts from yohimbe have been used in traditional medicine in west Africa as an aphrodisiac.

The drug can be taken orally to arouse sexual excitement and for erectile dysfunction (ED) by increasing blood flow and nerve impulses to the penis and/or vagina. It also helps to counteract the sexual side effects caused by medications for depression. It is available under several trade names including Aphrodyne and Yohimex. However, adverse side effects include increased heart rate, high blood pressure, dizziness, flushing of

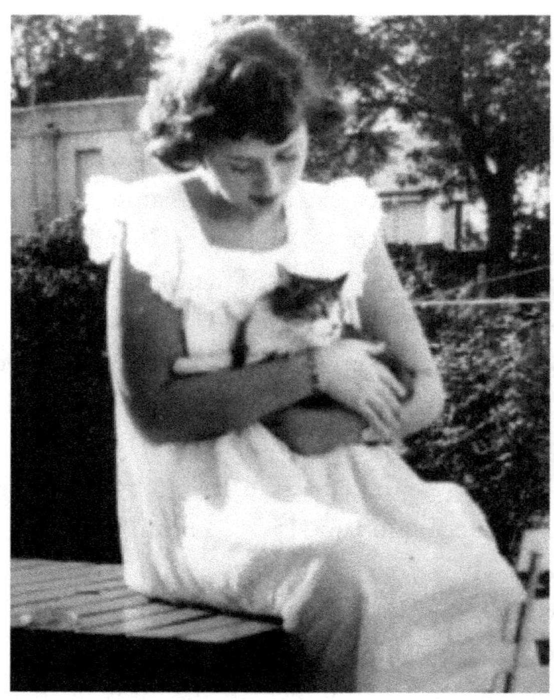

The mystery surrounding the deaths of Margaret Chandler and Dr Bogle has fascinated Australians for years. File picture courtesy of The Daily Telegraph.

the skin and nausea. There are recorded cases of a 69-year-old man dying during sexual intercourse after taking yohimbine and a 30-year-old woman found dead after consuming rauwolfia powder.

Could this have been the means that resulted in the deaths of Dr Gilbert Bogle and Margaret Chandler? I believe the police investigating the matter at the time were very close to the mark.

A similar case in Hong Kong was found four years later in 1967 by Dr Pang Teng Cheung, Director of Forensic Medicine, Hong Kong Police. He had uncovered the deaths of a couple that showed the same strange features as Dr Bogle and Mrs Chandler. This couple had died after taking yohimbine. There were rumours that Dr Bogle was suffering from sexual difficulties, a terrible development for someone with his excessive desires. Could his new lover have tried this exotic drug, with fatal results? Mrs

Chandler was a registered nurse. Hence, she would have had access to various drugs, including yohimbine, at that time.

Police initially suspected poisoning of the couple and I have to agree. Why did the couple choose the riverside location, even with a roll of carpet to lie on, when a vacant bedroom was to be had with a comfortable bed that had been offered? It appeared their lust for each other had eclipsed other rationale, and it was most likely drug enhanced, if not induced.

Many theories were published at the time, some quite outrageous and I'm sure were just to sell papers, so, I will not give them mention these. However, another plausible theory which surfaced quite recently was presented by Peter Butt in his book titled, *Who Killed Dr Bogle and Mrs Chandler?*, where he suggested that the two deaths were caused by accidental hydrogen sulphide poisoning from the contaminated Lane Cove River.

This was followed up by a documentary shown on the ABC in September 2006. I have to agree up to a point; hydrogen sulphide (commonly known as 'rotten egg' gas) is very toxic and is comparable to hydrogen cyanide in toxicity. I had a case where two sewerage workers had climbed down an inspection shaft and succumbed to the gas that had accumulated at the bottom. Their attempted rescuer almost died too, trying to save them. Also, eruptions of noxious gas from river beds (up-wellings) and other water sources such as lakes, have occurred around the world. For example, on 21 August 1986, a deadly, cloudy mixture of carbon dioxide and watery mist arose violently from Lake Nyos, Cameroon in west Africa. As the lethal cloud swept down adjacent valleys, it killed over 1700 people, thousands of cattle and native wildlife including, birds and animals. But the most important feature of this awful incident was that it not only killed humans, it also killed much wildlife too.

In the Bogle-Chandler scenario, no other obvious dead wildlife were found on the riverbanks, apart from some dead fish found in the river.

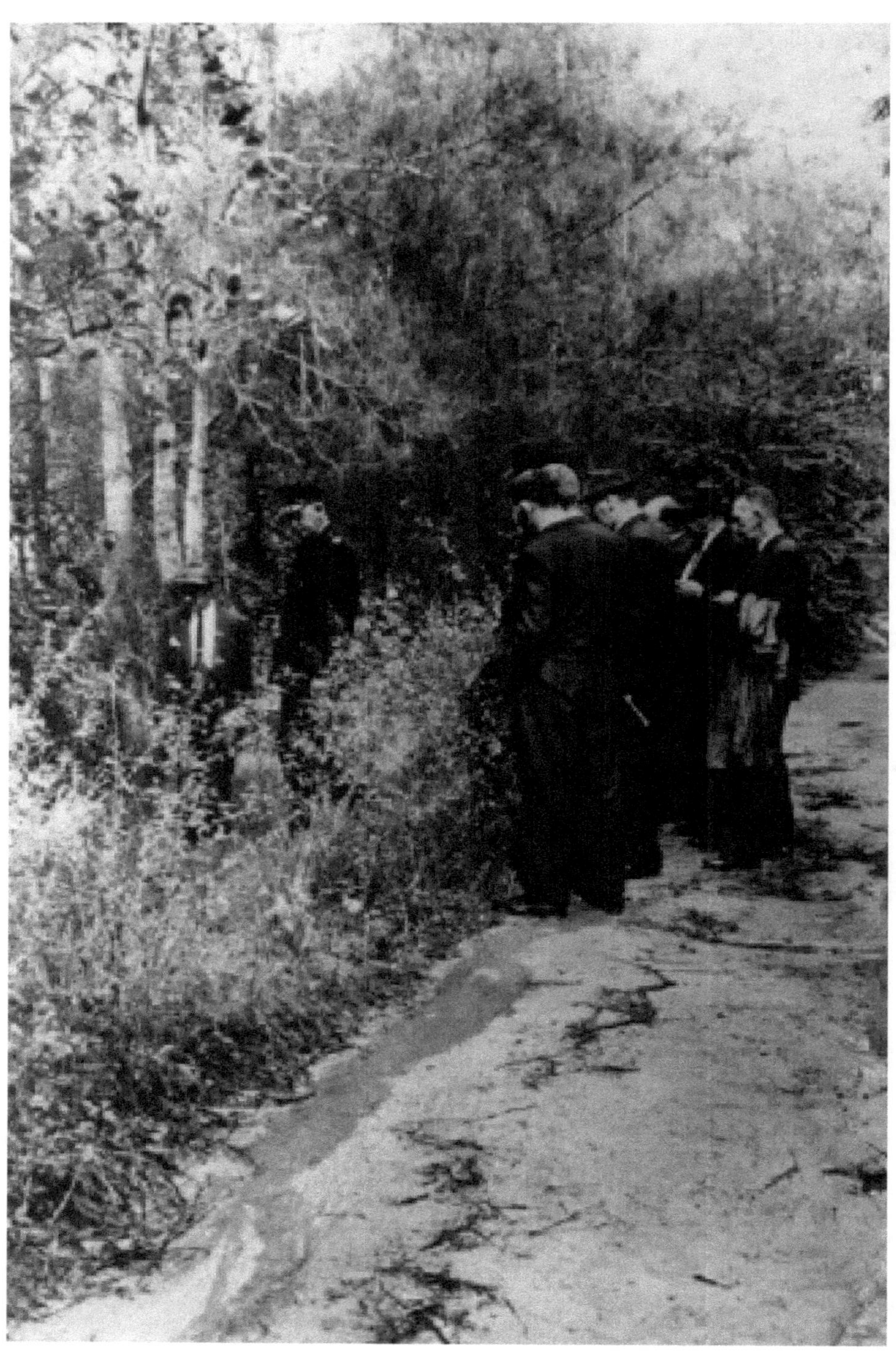

If there was an 'eruption' of hydrogen sulphide from the river, as has been suggested, why wasn't the area 'littered' with dead animals such as rabbits, foxes and possums? None were reported apart from a 'smelly dog' who had ventured into the area – and was still alive!

Given it was a New Year's Eve party, and the free and easy relationships that existed at the time amongst this group of people, I believe it was most likely a drink-spiking prank that went terribly wrong – or one of the participants in the sexual tryst wanted to 'turn the other on' but used too much of the drug to their terrible detriment.

I believe the latter was the more likely scenario.

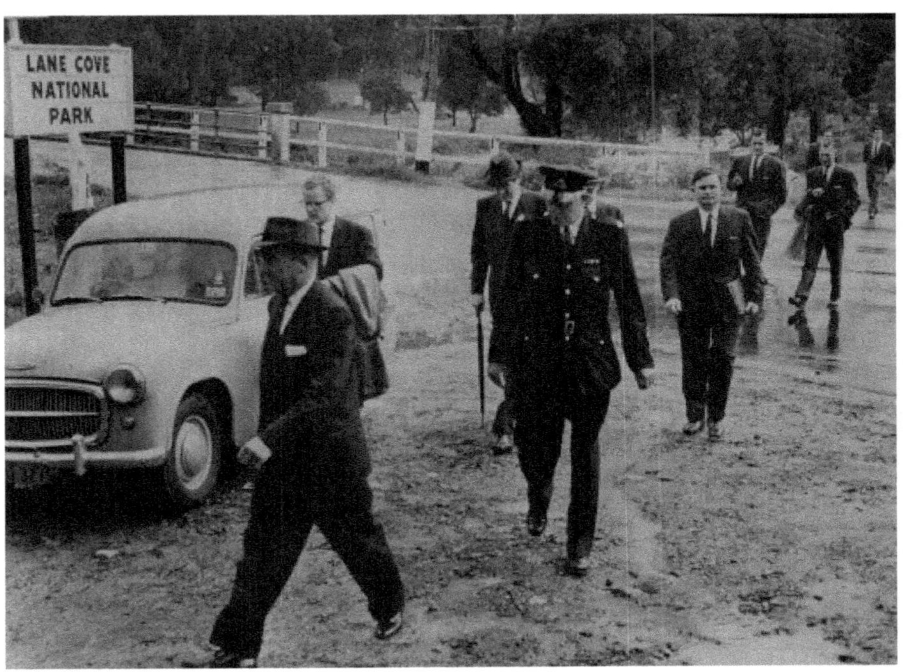

Officials arrive to examine the scene where the bodies were found during the inquest into the deaths. File picture courtesy of The Daily Telegraph.

Opposite: Police at the scene after the bodies were found.
File picture courtesy of The Daily Telegraph.

Colchicine Poisonings: The Dark Side of an Ancient Medicine

'Poison is in everything, and no thing is without poison. The dosage makes it either a poison or a remedy.'
– Paracelsus

Colchicine is a naturally occurring alkaloid derivative present in the corm and seeds of the meadow saffron (*Colchicum autumnale*) and in the flame or glory lily (*Gloriosa superba*) belonging to the plant family Colchicaceae. The plants are tuberous rooted deciduous perennials and have been used to treat gout for centuries. Generally, the colchicine content is higher in cultivated plants than the naturally grown plants, and the seed contains more colchicine than the tubers. The toxic properties of the plants have been known since the late third century BC, according to Pedanius Dioscorides (40–90 AD) who was a Greek physician, botanist, pharmacologist and author of *De Materia Medica*.

★

Medicinal preparations of the colchicine plants, in particular, *Colchicum autumnale*, have been prescribed for patients with joint pain since as early as the sixth century AD. Colchicine and colchicum preparations have been used for the relief of pain in acute gout, said to be even as early as some 50 centuries ago in ancient Egypt. Benjamin Franklin is apparently credited with introducing this therapy into the United States in 1763 for the treatment of this painful complaint. The drug was also reported to be effective for the treatment of periodic peritonitis (inflammation of the peritoneum, the tissue that lines the inner wall of the abdomen) and familial Mediterranean fever.

Unfortunately, the drug has a narrow therapeutic range; in toxic levels, colchicine can disproportionately affect rapidly dividing cells and have substantial effects on multiple organ systems. The total amount of colchicine required to relieve an acute attack of gout is between 3 and 6 milligrams. However, a total of 6 milligrams (10 tablets) should not be exceeded during a single course of treatment.

When orally ingested, colchicine is rapidly absorbed from the gastrointestinal tract and passed onto the liver, where it is metabolised via deacetylation and demethylation. Essentially, it is detoxified through the liver to innocuous substances. Large amounts of drug and metabolites are excreted into the bile and via the blood, into the intestinal tract, resulting in an enterohepatic circulation. Unfortunately, it is this rapid circulation that most likely accounts for the gastrointestinal side-effects observed, namely, severe abdominal pain, nausea, vomiting and diarrhoea characteristic of colchicine poisoning. Symptoms set in only after an interval of three to six hours, even with large doses, resulting in an ascending paralysis of the central nervous system (CNS), with death occurring from respiratory arrest generally within one to two days.

Not a nice way to end one's life.

However, I have had two cases where two depressed men chose this way to end their lives by ingesting excessive amounts of a colchicine preparation.

The first case was of a 61-year-old single man found dead beside his bed at 12.15 pm by a Meals on Wheels service worker. Beside the body was found a quantity of tablets and three bottles labelled 'Serepax' (a preparation containing oxazepam, a sedative), along with 'Prednisone' and 'Colchicine', the latter two bottles were empty. On a cupboard nearby there was a glass mug containing an amber-coloured liquid. It was later identified as being beer that contained a large quantity of white sediment. The deceased gentleman had been treated for scleroderma (chronic hardening and thickening of the skin) and had been recently released from hospital. Clearly, he had not been sufficiently counselled over his condition.

His body was conveyed to the morgue where an autopsy revealed a massive oedema and moderate congestion of his lungs. The bronchi, larynx and trachea contained a copious amount of mucopurulent secretion (a mixture of mucus and pus). The trachea and bronchial mucosa were moderately congested. Examination of his gastrointestinal tract revealed the oesophagus was thickened in the lower part and the mucosa appeared to be slightly sclerosed (hardened). The stomach contained about 400 millilitres of recently eaten food, indicating death was relatively fast. Liver, bile and stomach samples were collected for toxicological analysis.

A toxicological analysis of the thick white sediment in the glass mug revealed the presence of prednisone, colchicine and its decomposition product, lumicolchicine. The liver sample taken at a post-mortem was found to contain colchicine 0.1 milligrams per 100 milligrams of tissue, while the stomach contents contained 3 milligrams of colchicine, along with its decomposition product, lumicolchicine, and the bile was found to contain colchicine 0.32 milligrams per 100 millilitres of fluid.

In the second case, a 23-year old single unemployed man swallowed 25 to 50 milligrams of colchicine in tablet form (Colgout) with suicidal intent. As a result of this consumption he became ill and contacted his mother by telephone to get an ambulance. A short time later, his mother found him unconscious in his flat.

She promptly called an ambulance and he was taken to the nearest hospital. Unfortunately, despite the best efforts of the medical staff, the young man suffered a major cardiac arrest and died two days later.

His body was transferred to the morgue where an autopsy revealed a marked oedema of his lungs, with his respiratory passages containing frothy, bloodstained mucus. Examination of his gastrointestinal tract revealed marked para-oesophageal haemorrhage. The stomach contained some bloodstained fluid, and a few small haemorrhages were present in the gastric mucosa. Haemorrhages were also present in the mucosa and the wall of the small intestine in a number of places.

The poor fellow would have suffered a very difficult death.

A toxicological analysis was carried out on the liver, urine and stomach. The liver sample taken post-mortem was found to contain a colchicine breakdown product, colchiceine (des-methyl colchicine) 0.33 milligrams per 100 milligrams of tissue, while the stomach contents contained traces of lumicolchicine, and the urine was found to contain colchicine 1.25 milligrams per 100 millilitres of fluid.

It would appear that both men were aware of the toxic nature of colchicine. Suicide was achieved by consuming many times the lethal limit. In the first case described, the 61-year-old, chose a rather unusual method of consuming his poison, using beer as a 'chaser'. He evidently also thought that a large quantity of prednisone added to the drink would be effective. Maybe, but it was in a way he could not have imagined. He didn't suffer from the no-doubt painful haemorrhages the young man did, probably due to its anti-inflammatory properties.

After consuming a large quantity of the tablets, the 23-year-old man apparently had second thoughts about suicide as he began to feel the toxic effects set in. This particular case was toxicologically unusual because the colchicine was present in the hydrolysed form, colchiceine, possibly because of the prolonged period between consumption of the drug and death.

Apart from natural sources as described earlier, colchicine is generally not readily available except on prescription for the treatment of gout and other ailments such as periodic peritonitis. It is not often used in suicide, and occasionally poisonings occur through 'therapeutic misadventures'. The prolonged toxic effects, gastrointestinal disturbances and other effects, if known, would probably act as deterrents.

The use of colchicine in homicide is quite rare, making the next two cases notable. Neither of the two persons affected were taking the drug for therapeutic purposes.

The next two cases of the drug are from two different sources, firstly, *Gloriosa superba*, the well-known Asia glory or superb lily, which is a tropical climbing plant that produces a beautiful, exotic flame-red flower. The second, another Western source of the drug colchicine, from the meadow saffron (*Colchicum autumnale*), a beautiful flower commonly known as the autumn crocus, or 'naked ladies' due to the flowers emerging without any vegetation around it.

These cases turned out to be far more complex than the ones I had to deal with!

The first case involved a 27-year-old Sri Lankan man who was conveyed to the General Hospital Chilaw, Sri Lanka, suffering from profuse diarrhoea and vomiting, apparently after drinking a brew of coriander tea. This is a traditional Ayurvedic medicine treatment for the common cold, which had been prepared for him by his sister-in-law. The patient developed the symptoms some two hours after consuming the brew, during which time other family members noticed that the sister-in-law had slipped away. Suspicious, they examined the contents of the teapot. As expected, there were the coriander seeds, but there was something else; the pot also contained different seeds, which they soon realised were *Gloriosa* or flame lily seeds.

To the untrained eye, the seeds look very similar. However, the flame lily seeds were known to be available in the house as the young man worked on a farm that cultivated the *Gloriosa* vine, and on occasion brought some seeds home. Curious, his wife somewhat gamely tasted a small amount of the remaining brew in the tea pot and subsequently developed nausea and vomiting. In the meantime, the patient developed shock, respiratory distress and required ventilation and so was moved to the intensive care unit of the hospital. His total hospital stay was 15 days during which time he developed generalised alopecia (loss of hair). With appropriate medical treatment, he fully recovered from the acute toxicity.

However, without the patient's background and assistance from his family, this case could have been easily misdiagnosed as a severe case of food poisoning. Colchicine poisoning would not have been suspected until he developed the generalised alopecia. By then it would have been too late.

As there was reasonable suspicion that it was homicidal poisoning, the judicial medical consultant and the police were notified to proceed with a medico-legal investigation. During this time the patient admitted he had taken *Gloriosa* or flame lily seeds from his workplace, where the plants were grown for harvest and export of the seeds. A toxicological analysis of his gastric lavage samples revealed the presence of colchicine.

In this case, *Gloriosa* or flame lily seeds added to a coriander seed tea, were used in an attempted homicide – and almost succeeded, but for the awareness of a family member. Boiling water would have released the colchicine from the seeds into the tea thus preparing the potentially deadly brew.

The next case was quite different, but involved the same drug.

Mary Yoder, a 60-year-old New York chiropractor was attending to her patients one Sunday on 22 July 2015 at her Whitesboro medical practice, which she and her husband owned and successfully ran for more than 30 years. On this particular Sunday afternoon, Ms Yoder became ill after seeing a number of patients throughout the day and went home earlier than usual at about 4.30 pm.

Ms Yoder, generally a picture of health, was now suffering from severe vomiting attacks and diarrhoea. She tried to sleep it off when she got home, but by the following morning her symptoms were worsening. Her husband Bill, now clearly concerned, took her to the emergency unit of St Luke's hospital where the doctors ran a series of tests to work out what was making her so sick. Twenty-four hours had now passed since Ms Yoder first became sick.

The doctors were still at a loss as to what was happening to their patient and admitted her to the ICU of the hospital. Unfortunately, even here she continued to deteriorate and the following morning she suffered her first heart attack, followed by seven more. It is amazing she survived that many heart attacks. But another one in the afternoon was one too many, and sadly it took her life.

Due to the circumstances of Mary Yoder's death a post-mortem was carried out the following day. The examination revealed her tissues and organs were undergoing a condition known as apoptosis, or cell death due to inhibited cell division. It was a clear sign of poisoning – this was not a natural death.

But what poison was causing this condition? After the PM, the medical examiner's office sent her samples to another laboratory, NMS Labs in Pennsylvania, for further testing. Initial testing for common poisons including arsenic and cyanide proved negative.

Two months passed, and then the chemists got a positive result. Ms Yoder's blood sample was found to contain colchicine. Then further testing of her gastric content sample revealed high levels of colchicine.

It was now known that Mary Yoder had died from a lethal dose of colchicine, most likely orally ingested.

So, the drug that killed her was identified, it was then up to the investigators to find out how it got in her body: was it an accident, suicide or murder? Mary Yoder's medical practice included a belief in holistic medicine and herbal supplements, even growing some of her own herbs in her beloved home garden. Investigators thought it prudent to check out her garden. But no plants belonging to the plant family Colchicaceae, such as meadow saffron were found. It was also known she endorsed supplements, so a search was instigated to see if there was any contamination of the supplements. These were collected and subjected to extensive testing. The results revealed no garden source of the drug. No contamination of the supplements used in her practice. And suicide was ruled out after speaking to family and friends.

Mary Yoder's death was no mishap.

That now left the unsettling option: murder. But who would want to murder her and for what reason? However, on the day Ms Yoder became ill, her husband, Bill, who was often at her side, wasn't around. Curiously, not long after Mary Yoder died, he was apparently dating her older sister, Kathleen Richmond. It was not a good look, and the police began to suspect him as the person responsible for Mary's death.

Then the authorities began to receive anonymous letters claiming to know who poisoned Mary Yoder. Further, they implicated Mary Yoder's son, Adam Yoder, and also identified the poison used, colchicine. However, Dr Bill Yoder wasn't entirely ruled out of the investigation, as they turned their attention onto Adam. He was subsequently questioned about the letters and their contents, suggesting there was evidence in his car that police would have been interested in.

Sure enough, the sheriff's deputies checked out Adam's car, a Jeep Wrangler, and found under the passenger seat the evidence described in the letter. There they found a bottle of colchicine, a cardboard wrapper and a receipt detailing the purchase and, probably most damaging of all, an email address similar to that Mr Yoder had describing the transaction.

It appeared the police had their prime suspect.

What they needed now was to corroborate their findings and interview witnesses. The obvious one, was Kaitlyn Conley, Adam's, on-and-off girlfriend. She also worked for the Mary and Bill Yoder at their chiropractic business for several years on the front desk, both as a receptionist and office manager. The investigating detectives thought that if anything was going on between Adam Yoder and his mother, Ms Conley may be able to provide some answers. Initially, the police were expecting her to provide some evidence regarding Dr Yoder. Instead, Adam Yoder was implicated. She was pointing the finger at her former boyfriend!

Further, the State Police Forensics Laboratory had tested the anonymous letters for DNA. There was female DNA detected under the stamp of the letter. A DNA sample was subsequently provided by Ms Conley which matched that found under the stamp. Kaitlyn Conley offered the explanation that she worked in the office and generally pre-stamped the envelopes. So far, so good. However, detectives decided to take another look at the evidence collected from Adam Yoder's Jeep Wrangler. Along with the bottle of colchicine tablets was the receipt and an email address attached to the transaction. Adam was questioned by detectives about this and he said that it was similar to one he had but that it was not his account. The email address was traced to two places, one at Kaitlyn Conley's home and the other on her cell phone.

It looked like Adam Yoder was being framed for the murder.

It appeared the 'evidence' in Adam's car was deliberately planted there. The detectives interviewed Ms Conley again and she continued to implicate Adam Yoder. Given the detection of her DNA on the stamp of the anonymous letter, she was asked whether she wrote the letter. Surprisingly, she admitted to writing the letter. From that point, Adam Yoder was no longer the prime suspect, that role was shifted to Kaitlyn Conley, 23. She was arrested and charged with second-degree murder for the death of Mary Yoder.

But why was Ms Yoder murdered? What was the motive?

The matter initially went before the Oneida County courthouse in the quiet upstate New York city of Utica. The defence barrister for Kaitlyn Conley, Mr Christopher Pelli, said that the case was 'entirely about motive'. He further alleged that only one person had the motive and knowledge to kill Mary Yoder declaring, 'the decedent's husband' Bill Yoder, the man who went missing on the day Mary Yoder became sick. Mr Pelli then speculated that Mary's daily protein shake was spiked with the drug before work, suggesting that was why he was not at the office that day. Motive, he further suggested, was through an alleged illicit affair with Mary's sister, Kathleen ('Kathy') Richmond.

Curiously, this claim was supported by Mary Yoder's sister, Janine King. But the prosecutor, Ms Laurie Lisi, disagreed and said that Dr Bill Yoder had nothing to do with the murder. It was all Kaitlyn and the motive for the murder was 'pure and simple': revenge. It was put before the court that essentially, after Adam Yoder broke up with Kaitlyn Conley, she felt like a woman scorned and she wanted to get back at Adam by killing his mother.

Kaitlyn Conley had clearly built up a fair amount of trust between Mary's own sisters, who disagreed with the prosecutions findings, Janine King saying, 'We thought she was being framed.'

Then, after some three weeks of testimony and five days of deliberations, the defence had created enough doubt to leave the jurors 'hopelessly deadlocked'. Such that the judge was forced to declare a mistrial. An initial success for the defence.

However, the prosecutors did not allow the charges to be dropped, and five months later Kaitlyn Conley was back on trial for murder.

Kaitlyn's family then hired a new barrister for her second trial, Mr Frank Policelli. He chose to take a different tactic. While accepting the fact that Mary Yoder died from colchicine poisoning, he accused Mary's son and Kaitlyn's former boyfriend of carrying out the deed. This was further supported by Mary's sister Janine King who was reported to say, 'Adam is a troubled person and Mary and he had had a falling out.' This view was supported by Mary's nephew, David King, who shared accommodation with Adam during the time he was dating Kaitlyn Conley and spoke of their stormy relationship. He was asked, 'Do you think Katie was a victim of domestic violence at the hands of Adam, allegedly?'

'I do,' replied Mr King.

The tactic now was to suggest it was Adam, not Kaitlyn, who was seeking revenge, such that he set out to implicate her in his mother's murder after she refused to get back together with him. To support this view, Ms Conley's defence entered into evidence text messages from Adam to Kaitlyn where he appears to want her back. One he allegedly wrote was, 'I miss you a lot. I'm thinking about you always.' There were other texts alluding to Kaitlyn's pregnancy to Adam and subsequent termination of the pregnancy.

Mr King said, 'He said he intended to marry her at one point.'

These texts from Adam Yoder appear to undermine the prosecution's case that Kaitlyn Conley killed Mary Yoder in revenge after Adam rejected her. Still, the prosecution had their doubts.

However, there was a significant change that prosecutors made between the two trials. Prosecutors added on the lesser charge of first-degree manslaughter for the jury to consider if they found Kaitlyn not guilty on the second-degree murder charge.

After weeks of testimony, the jurors began their deliberations. To help them reach a decision, they requested another look at the police interrogation video (known as an ERISP – Electronically Recorded Interview of a Suspected Person – in Australia). Here the detective asked why Adam would keep the incriminating colchicine tablets in his Jeep. Kaitlyn replied that he wanted to use it for someone else. Then contradicted herself by saying, guys don't use poison. The interviewing detective comments, 'A lot of them do.'

Kaitlyn then says, 'They say it's a lady's weapon.' It was a curious comment. And the jurors were beginning to doubt that Adam Yoder would have murdered his mother. Instead the prosecution's electronic evidence, along with searches and transactions recorded on Kaitlyn Conley's phone and computer were proving quite incriminating.

The prosecutor summed up, 'The evidence is clear and that the common denominator is the defendant, Kaitlyn Conley.'

Subsequently, Kaitlyn Conley, by then 24 years old, was found guilty of first-degree manslaughter. After a number of appeals, some from unexpected quarters. It was time for the victim-impact statements. The most damaging was from Kaitlyn's former boyfriend, Adam Yoder, who said he hated her because she murdered his mother. Then Mary Yoder's husband of 40 years, testified that Kaitlyn Conley sought to get even with his son by murdering his mother. However, there's no mention about framing him for the crime to boot!

Predictably, Kaitlyn still declares her innocence, and then thanks her family, friends and strangers who supported her.

Eventually it was up to Judge Michael Dwyer to announce Kaitlyn Conley's fate saying, 'The evidence presented at the trial indicates that Ms Conley was the only person at that time that knew why this was happening and how her life was going to end. It will be the sentence of this court as to the defendant's conviction for manslaughter in the first degree that she will be sentenced to a 23-year determinant sentence in state prison.'

After two trials and many weeks of testimony, this strange case finally came to a close.

But as with most crimes, it was the family who were left mourning the loss of one of their beloved members, and this is a life-long sentence.

The Aberdeen Butcher:
The Horrific Crimes of
Katherine Knight

'All evils are equal when they are extreme.'
– Pierre Corneille, **Horace**

This story takes place in Aberdeen, a small township situated in the midst of the fertile pastoral and agricultural countryside of New South Wales, Australia. The town is located on the side of a hill, alongside the Hunter River, between Muswellbrook and Scone on the New England Highway. It was named after Aberdeen, in Scotland, and is 273 kilometres north of Sydney. The 2006 census recorded its population as 1791.

The district around Aberdeen was once occupied by the Wanaruah Aboriginal people. Because so few written records of Aboriginal Australia were kept, it's difficult to determine their lifestyle in pre-colonial Australia. However, it is known that the Wanaruah had trade and ceremonial links with another Aboriginal tribe, the Kamilaroi, who may also have occupied the area. They were peaceful people who lived off the land, their favourite meal being goanna, along with kangaroo and assorted wildlife, which was roasted over campfire coals after being gutted and stuffed with grass. A traditional aboriginal feast for this area.

Many years later, the colonists moved in and established an abattoir to cater for the processing of fat beef cattle that were then raised on the rich pastures in the surrounding areas of the newly established township. That and the mining industry became the mainstays of Aberdeen. However, the abattoir was the main employer, providing work for more than 400 people from the town and surrounding areas, such as Scone.

It was in this setting, that one of the most gruesome murders in Australia's history took place.

★

Katherine Mary Knight was born about half an hour after her fraternal twin sister, Joy Gwendoline, at Tenterfield Hospital in north-western New South Wales on 24 October 1955. Their father, Ken, was a skilled slaughterman, working at the local abattoir. He and his wife, Barbara, had eight children, six of whom were boys. It was a tough call supporting a family of that size, as Ken's wages had to stretch to feed ten people, seven days a week. Every meal had to count and Barbara's work was cut out with cooking, cleaning, sewing and raising the eight little ones. The previous night's lamb roast had to be turned into the following day's shepherd's pie and so on, with other offerings for the rest of week. All in all, a typical working Australian family of those times.

Katherine was generally a pleasant girl, and her red hair and freckles earned her the nickname of 'the speckled hen'. Very much a loner, with only a couple of friends, she spent a lot of time playing with her dolls. However, she loved animals, or at least pretty much any creature that was injured. Sadly, she wasn't allowed to have any pets because her father kept greyhounds and was afraid they would be eaten by the dogs, but undeterred, she still picked up injured strays, small birds and so on, took them home and nursed them back to health.

Unfortunately, that good nature started to dissipate as she got older, when she also started to experience extraordinary rages over relatively minor upsets. She began to savour the smells of the meat industry and developed a yearning to work at the abattoir like her father. When she left

Muswellbrook High School at the age of 15, supposedly almost illiterate, she landed a job as a cutter in a clothing factory. It wasn't exactly what she was looking for, and after a year she left and got a position at the abattoir, cutting up offal. She loved it, and her enthusiasm was eventually rewarded when she was promoted to boning and presented with her own set of butcher knives, which she proudly hung over her bed so that they, 'would always be handy if I needed them'. She was said to have been as raunchy and heartless as any male worker, and appeared to be quite proud of it. A tough woman in a tough environment.

In 1974, at the age of 18, she married 22-year-old co-worker David Stanford Kellett, a former railway worker turned slicer. The couple arrived at the marriage service on Katherine's motorcycle, with a very drunk Kellett on the pillion seat. Katherine's mother took him aside and warned, 'You better watch this one or she'll fucking kill you. Stir her up the wrong way or do the wrong thing and you're fucked. Don't ever think of playing up on her, she'll fucking kill you.' David just laughed it off, but Barbara wasn't joking, and it was said that Katherine tried to strangle him on their wedding night after he'd fallen asleep following several heavy bouts of sex.

Later on, David Kellett took another job at the abattoir – stunning pigs with a stun gun – which Katherine allegedly enjoyed watching.

Their first child, Melissa Ann, was born on 11 May 1976, but the marriage had become very shaky, and David had begun an affair with another Aberdeen woman. Unable to handle Katherine's moods and rages, he took off to Queensland with his now pregnant mistress. That relationship was doomed and ended soon after the birth of the child.

Katherine was devastated by David's desertion and took her rage out on their newborn daughter, leaving the two-month-old baby in the middle of a railway track to be killed by the next train. Fortunately, Ted Abrahams, a pensioner who lived in a small room on the ground floor of the Aberdeen Hotel, heard the baby crying. He'd been foraging along the top of an embankment near the tracks at the time, and rescued the child, just minutes before a train passed through.

Later that same day, Katherine grabbed an axe from a woodpile and started swinging it above her head and threatening people. She was apprehended by police and taken to St Elmo's Hospital in Tamworth for treatment, where she was subsequently discharged, with the doctors saying she was suffering from postnatal depression.

Soon after that, on Tuesday 3 August, Katherine slashed a young woman's face with a knife after the woman told her that Melissa was sick. She demanded that the poor woman take her to her husband. Having little option but to comply, the bleeding woman drove to the Bogas petrol station for petrol, but managed to escape. In the meantime, Katherine grabbed a little boy and threatened to slash him. When the police arrived, she was holding the child with one hand and a knife in the other. The two officers, choosing a less violent approach to defuse the situation, grabbed a couple of broomsticks and tried to knock the knife out of Katherine's hand, all the while telling her to drop the weapon. After prodding her several times with the broomsticks, she did and she was promptly arrested. The police then took her to a doctor in Muswellbrook, who issued a Schedule 2 under the Mental Health Act, and she was taken to Morisset Psychiatric Hospital for treatment, where she was diagnosed with personality disorder.

While she was in the hospital, her three-month-old baby daughter was looked after by her grandparents, Barbara and Ken. Katherine was subsequently discharged after six days into the care and custody of Jean Dobson (David Keller's mother), and soon after, Katherine, David and their baby daughter Melissa got back together, living in a rented bungalow in Woodridge, Queensland, where David drove trucks and Katherine took up a job boning carcasses at the Dinmore Abattoir, in nearby Ipswich.

Despite the many difficulties experienced in the marriage, the couple did what warring spouses often do, they had another baby. Natasha Maree Kellett was born on 6 March 1980 in Nambour hospital.

Four years later, Katherine and David again separated. Katherine moved in with her parents in Aberdeen before renting a house in Muswellbrook and taking up work at her former place of employment, the Aberdeen abattoir. Her estranged husband moved to Alice Springs, where he found work as a trucker. Although they were separated, he was still a doting father, sending his girls presents and cards at Christmas and flowers on their birthdays. But they never knew about them because Katherine disposed of them before the girls were able to receive them.

In 1986, Katherine met a 38-year-old miner, David Saunders, at a local hotel. He was a good-natured hard drinker. Katherine turned on the charm, and they soon hit it off. A few months later, he moved in with her and her two daughters.

But it wasn't long before the jealous rages began and she threw him out of the house. He then moved back to his apartment in Scone, and after a time, Katherine would go around and beg him to come back. He always returned. It appeared her voracious sexual appetite overrode any other concerns. In May 1987, she slit the throat of his two-month-old dingo pup with one of her boning knives before going on to bash him on the head with a frying pan until he was unconscious. Those acts of violence were to show Saunders what would happen if he had an affair. And he hadn't even contemplated it!

In June 1988, Katherine gave birth to her third daughter. With a growing family, David Saunders decided to move out of their housing commission house and get one of their own. The house was paid off the following year when Katherine's worker's compensation (from a previous back injury received at the abattoir) came through. Meanwhile, Katherine had developed a macabre interest in dead animals and decorated their cottage with a variety of animal skins, cow and sheep skulls, water buffalo and steer horns, deer antlers, rusted animal traps, old fashioned fur wraps and assorted stuffed animals and birds. It was a real museum of death.

Her rages hadn't stopped either. After yet another argument, she hit Saunders over the head with an iron and stabbed him with a pair of scissors. And in an act of real spite, she cut up all his clothes. Unsurprisingly, he left her, but when he returned later to see his daughter, he discovered that Katherine had taken out an appended violence order (AVO). She'd told the police that he'd been abusing her and they believed her. David Saunders then went away for good, not realising exactly how kind fate had been to him.

In 1990, Katherine met up with John 'Chillo' Chillingworth, a 43-year-old former abattoir co-worker, at the local hotel. At the time, he was unaware of her violent moods, but his friends warned him that she was bad news. Their relationship, while stormy, produced a son, Eric, who was born in 1991. But Katherine started having an affair with another Aberdeen local, John 'Pricey' Price, and the relationship with John Chillingworth ended after three years. Although he didn't know it at the time, he was very fortunate to be free of Katherine and was able to get on with his own life. However, the same could not be said of John Price.

When he became entangled with Katherine, he was already the father of three children. Recently amicably separated from his wife, Colleen, he was feeling lonely and so quickly fell for Katherine's charms. It was 1993. They were both 38 and Pricey was totally smitten by her. He was a very popular man, very likeable and very generous. It was said that 'he would give you his last two bob'. A top bloke.

He worked at the Howick Mines in Aberdeen, making a good living, and had a comfortable brick home in St Andrews Street, which had been left to him by his former wife, Colleen. In 1995, Katherine moved in with him. The house was quite luxurious compared to her 'dead animal museum' cottage and at first she treated him very well, as was her usual way, doing all the things that a loving wife does, and they also supposedly had quite a vigorous sex life. Happy days. But it didn't last. The honeymoon period ended and the drinking and insane violence began.

In 1998, Katherine decided she wanted some permanence in their relationship and wanted John to marry her. He refused, and in retaliation, she videotaped some items allegedly stolen from work and sent the tape to his boss. The items were only outdated medical kits that had been given to him by the storeman, but nevertheless, it cost Pricey his job, a position he'd held and loved for 17 years. He was devastated.

He promptly threw Katherine out of his home and she returned to her home in MacQueen Street. Pricey was now unemployed and lonely, and after a few months they resumed their relationship, although she didn't move back into his house. Pricey's friends were amazed that he'd taken her back after what the 'poisonous speckled hen' (a disparaging term now given to Katherine) had done to him. Laurie Lewis, one of his close friends, said he wanted nothing more to do with 'that woman'. Unfortunately for Pricey, that had a knock-on effect, because other people in his life would not associate with Katherine, including his children, Rosemary, Jackeline (Jackie) and Johnathon, which led to him becoming isolated to some extent. Not only did the reconciliation come at considerable cost, but the emotional scars would never heal. Pricey could forgive, but he couldn't forget, and so the arguments and fights resumed.

Fortunately, he landed another job a few months after being sacked from Howick Mines. It was with a company called Bowditch and Partners Earthmoving Pty Ltd, and his bosses soon recognised his skills with heavy machinery.

However, Katherine was still consumed with her irrational and venomous need for revenge and on 29 February 2000, she took a knife and stabbed him in the upper left chest, prompting him to take out an AVO against her to keep her away from him and his children. But so determined was she to up the ante, she just ignored it.

That same afternoon, Pricey said to his co-workers, somewhat prophetically, that if he didn't come into work the following day, it would be because Katherine had done him in. Concerned about the situation, his co-workers said that he shouldn't go home, but Pricey felt that if he didn't, she would kill his children.

In the meantime, and unknown to him, Katherine had sent the children away for a sleepover at a friend's place, so when Pricey arrived home, there was no-one there. After an evening watching television, he took a shower and went to bed. Katherine sneaked into his house and woke him just after 11 pm. She must have used all her feminine wiles because they had sex, after which he fell asleep.

A night of terror was about to begin.

Katherine had brought her butcher's knife with her, and it was within easy reach. The first blow was struck without warning, followed by several others to his naked chest. She was now doing what she had threatened many times before — she was murdering him. In stark terror and agony, Pricey leapt out of bed, running down the hallway with Katherine in relentless pursuit, all the time stabbing continuously at her mortally wounded victim. Blood from his numerous wounds stained the bedding, carpet and walls as he made a desperate attempt to escape. But the blade kept plunging into him. The pain must have been unbearable and with his lungs now badly damaged, he couldn't shout to raise the alarm. Amazingly, he clung to life, staggering to the front door and leaving a bloody hand print on the door frame. But he couldn't make it through and he was dragged back into the house where he collapsed. The stabbings continued and he slid down the wall of the entrance foyer, where he died. (An autopsy would later reveal that he'd been stabbed at least 37 times, in both the front and back of his body, with many of the wounds damaging vital organs.)

With Pricey dead, Katherine stripped off her bloodstained clothing and had a shower. Then she went into Aberdeen and at the ATM withdrew a sum of $500 at 2.32 am followed by a further sum of $500 at 2.35 am – a total of $1000, the maximum allowed at one drawing – from Pricey's account.

But her grisly night's work and revenge were still not complete.

At 6 am the following morning, a neighbour noticed that Pricey's white Ford Mondeo sedan was still in the driveway. That's so unlike Pricey, he thought. Normally, he'd have been away to work and he was known as being very punctual, so when he didn't arrive at Bowditch and Partners, his employer sent a fellow worker around to his house to see if he was okay. The neighbour and worker noticed Pricey's work boots were still lined up at the front door, as was his custom. Thinking that he may have overslept, they tried waking him by knocking on his bedroom window. It was then that they spotted blood stains on the front door and contacted the police. Sergeant Furlonger and Senior Constables Maude and Matthews arrived at the St Andrews Street property 25 minutes later, at 8.10 am. They tried the front and back doors, finding each to be locked, and used a crowbar to gain entry via the laundry door.

The police officers had decades of experience between them, but nothing could have prepared them for what they were about to witness.

Led by Sergeant Furlonger, they entered the premises with their weapons drawn. There was blood everywhere and a large pool of blood near the entrance foyer. Then what was thought to be a blanket hanging in a doorway arch leading into the lounge turned out to be, on closer inspection, John Price's exterior layer of skin hanging from a meat hook.

'Oh my God, she's skinned him!' one of the officers gasped.

It was a human pelt, expertly removed in one piece.

Moving further into the house, they found the victim's decapitated remains on the lounge room floor, near a small foyer leading to the front door. The body was raw and bloodless. Given the injuries and blood loss, that was hardly surprising. The left arm of John Price's body was draped over an empty 1.25-litre soft drink bottle and his legs were crossed. A butchers' knife was found close by. (Two more knives were later found in the kitchen.)

As the police officers moved through the house, they caught the smell of something that had been cooking coming from the kitchen. Further extreme horrors were to be revealed.

There was a large boiler pot, still warm, on the stove. On opening the lid, they saw John Price's skinned head, along with a quantity of vegetables. After Katherine had decapitated him, she'd cooked parts of his body, serving up the meat with a variety of vegetables, including baked potatoes and gravy, in three settings at the dinner table. She'd also prepared notes alongside the plates, each one having the name of one of his children written on it. Many of the surfaces were heavily bloodstained. A third piece of cooked meat (later identified to be from John Price's left buttock) was found in the backyard. (It has been speculated that Katherine Knight had attempted to eat it but had been unable to do so and tossed it onto the back lawn. However, that has never been established to any degree of certainty.)

A further bloodstained note was found on a small display cabinet in the lounge room, near the hanging skin. It read: 'Now play with little Johns dick John Price. Time got back Johnathon for rapping [raping] my douter [daughter]. You to Ross and Little John.' (The words were found to be nonsense.)

The police officers then checked the bathroom and found it was empty, save for a black nightie tossed carelessly over the side of the bath. It was heavily bloodstained with what appeared to be flecks of meat adhering to the cloth.

Then they heard a loud snoring sound coming from the main bedroom and looked through the door. The light switch was bloodstained and the sleeping body of Katherine Knight was lying fully clothed on the double bed. With some difficulty, she was aroused and handcuffed. At 8.25 am, an ambulance was summoned, along with police backup, and the house and surrounding area were declared to be a crime scene.

Katherine Knight was sitting on the ground behind a police vehicle when the ambulance arrived. She was dishevelled, her face was flushed and her speech was slurred. Upon examination, the ambulance crew formed the opinion that she'd taken an excessive amount of medication. (Empty packets of medication were later found on the kitchen bench of the house.) She was loaded into the ambulance, which left at 9.16 am, arriving at Muswellbrook Hospital eight minutes later. She was later transferred to the accident and emergency department, where she was placed under the care of medical staff. A blood sample was taken as standard procedure.

The subsequent toxicology report revealed that the blood sample contained fluvoxamine 0.22 milligrams per litre and promethazine 0.21 milligrams per litre. No alcohol was detected.

Fluvoxamine is a serotonin re-uptake inhibitor (SNRI) antidepressant that can result in dizziness and drowsiness. It's available under the trade name Luvox, and is used to treat emotional depression. The therapeutic range for this drug is 0.05 to 0.25 milligrams per litre of blood, meaning the level found in Katherine Knight's blood was towards the top end.

Promethazine is a phenothiazine-type antihistamine that can also result in dizziness and drowsiness, and would therefore exacerbate the effects of fluvoxamine. It's available under several trade names, including Phenergan, which is used to treat hayfever and allergy symptoms. The therapeutic range for this drug is 0.1 to 0.4 milligrams per litre of blood, so the level found in Katherine Knight's blood was mid-range.

Neither of the drugs were in the toxic range, but the two together resulted in Knight being found in a deep sleep. The outcome could have been quite different if she'd also consumed an appreciable quantity of alcohol in addition to the medication, but as it was, she was able to sleep it off and was not in any danger.

I found from earlier research that in most drug overdoses involving promethazine only, the levels were either very high (greater than 2 milligrams per litre — ten times more than that found in Katherine's blood), or another central nervous system depressant, such as oxazepam (Serepax) or alcohol, was present, and sometimes both.

Detective Sergeant Bob Wells and Detective Senior Constable Peter Muscio from the Maitland crime scene team were tasked with further investigations into John Price's gruesome murder, and on 6 March 2000, after the alleged suicide attempt, Katherine Knight was formally charged with the murder at Maitland District Hospital. She'd been placed in the psychiatric ward, where psychiatrists had assessed her mental state, concluding that she'd been sane when committing her heinous crimes.

Katherine Knight's defence counsel initially applied for the charge of murder to be reduced to one of manslaughter. Not unsurprisingly, it was rejected and Katherine was arraigned to appear before the court on 2 February 2001. She entered a plea of not guilty. The trial was initially set for 23 July but was postponed due to the illness of her counsel and given a new date of 15 October.

When the trial began, Justice Barry O'Keefe (jokingly known as the Mild One, as he was the brother of rocker, Johnny O'Keefe, the Wild One) offered the 60 jury prospects the option of being excused from duty due to the graphic nature of the evidence. Five accepted. Several more declined after the witness list had been read out.

The defence attorneys for Katherine Knight then spoke to the judge, who adjourned proceedings until the following day. When the trial commenced the next morning, Katherine Knight, surprisingly, pleaded guilty, and so the jury was dismissed. The plea saved John Price's family and a number of witnesses the ordeal of going through a lengthy traumatic trial.

In spite of that and the fact that Katherine's legal team had planned to defend her by claiming amnesia and dissociation, Justice O'Keefe ordered a psychiatric assessment to establish whether Katherine Knight understood the consequences of a guilty plea and whether she was fit to make such a plea. Although admitting her guilt, Katherine still refused to take responsibility for her very savage actions, and she was held in custody.

Several forensic psychiatrists, including Dr Robert Delaforce, determined that she'd been totally sane when she committed the crimes. He concluded, 'What she did on the night was part of her personality, her nature, herself, but it is not a feature of borderline personality disorder, it is not even significantly connected.'

On Thursday 8 November 2001, 618 days after the murder of John Price, his family returned to court, hoping that justice would prevail at the sentencing. Justice O'Keefe strode into the courtroom at 11 am. He had much to consider. There was no doubt that the barbaric murder fell into the worst case category, and under section 23A of the *Crimes Act 1900*, he had a choice of either sending Katherine to prison for the term of her natural life or he could grant her mercy and impose a long fixed sentence.

He began to read from his lengthy judgment, reiterating what had occurred on or about 29 February 2000. He described the manner in which John Price had died, which proved to be very hard for his children, who broke down, with one daughter having to leave the courtroom to compose herself. Then he moved on to Katherine's attempted suicide, saying it hadn't appeared genuine, quoting as evidence the relevant parts of the toxicology report that showed the blood levels of the drugs detected had been within therapeutic limits. He also noted that Katherine would have required a steady hand and much skill to remove the skin from John Price's deceased body in one piece, which included his head, face, nose, neck, torso, genitals and legs.

As for mercy, Justice O'Keefe said, 'The prisoner, Katherine Mary Knight, does not qualify for mercy. She engaged in cruel, vicious behaviour to Mr Price. She showed him no mercy. She has not expressed any contrition or remorse. If released, she poses a serious threat to the security of society. I'm satisfied beyond any doubt that such a murder was premeditated. I'm further satisfied in the same way that not only did she plan the murder, but she also enjoyed the horrific acts which followed in its wake as part of a ritual of dead and defilement.'

His Honour continued, 'The things which she did after the death of Mr Price indicate cognition, volition, calm and skill. I am satisfied beyond reasonable doubt that her evil actions were playing out of her resentments arising out of her rejection by Mr Price, her impending expulsion from Mr Price's home, which he wanted to retain for his children.

'As I have said, the prisoner showed no mercy whatsoever to Mr Price. The last minutes of his life must have been a time of abject terror for him, as they were a time of utter enjoyment for her. At no time did the prisoner express any regret for what she had done or any remorse for having done it; not even through the surrogacy of counsel. Her attitude in that regard is consistent with her general approach to the many acts of violence which she has engaged in against her various partners.'

Justice O'Keefe addressed the court for over an hour and said in his concluding comments, 'The only appropriate penalty for the prisoner is life imprisonment and that parole should never be considered for her.'

He then looked up from his judgment and asked Katherine Knight to stand before delivering the judgment that John Price's family were anxious to hear.

'Katherine Mary Knight, you have pleaded guilty to, and been convicted of, the murder of John Charles Thomas Price at Aberdeen in the State of New South Wales, on or about 29th February, 2000. In respect of that crime, I sentence you to imprisonment for life.'

She was led her away to the cells below the courtroom to await her final transport to Mulawa Women's Correctional Centre, where she would begin the rest of her life in prison.

She made history by becoming the first woman in Australia to be jailed for the term of her natural life.

Someone once said that the way to measure a man and how he led his life was at his funeral. I'm not so sure about that, given the lavish funerals that well-known gangsters have had at their deaths. But in John Price's case, I have to agree. He was a decent, hardworking Australian who loved his women, his kids, his mates and his beer, and very much in that order!

Pricey was truly a rough diamond, and as a result it was standing room only at St Alban's Anglican Church, Muswellbrook on 10 March 2000. Many others were unable to get a place in the church, and had to listen to the service outside.

When Pricey was alive, he was known as a top bloke, and that's exactly what he was. It showed at his funeral with the hundreds of people who came to pay their respects. His best friend, Laurie Lewis, and his two previous bosses, Geoffrey Bowditch and Peter Cairnes, delivered moving eulogies before the congregation. After the church service, the funeral cortege made its way along the New England Highway to the Aberdeen cemetery, where he was finally laid to rest.

In June 2006, Katherine Knight appealed her life sentence, claiming that the mutilation of John Price's body after his death was not relevant to the seriousness of the offence and that she hadn't received an adequate discount for her guilty plea. However, in September, justices Peter McClellan, Michael Adams and Megan Latham dismissed the appeal in the New South Wales Court of Criminal Appeal.

Justice Adams said the mutilation of the body was closely associated with the murder such that 'it must be regarded as an integral part of the killing itself. It demonstrates the extraordinary extent of the applicant's brutality.'

Justice McClellan commented, 'This was a violent and cruel crime during which the deceased must have suffered extreme trauma. The crime was the product of a violent personality intent upon claiming the life of her de facto in a relationship which was plainly failing. The psychiatric evidence indicates that her personality is unlikely to change in the future, and if released, she would be likely to inflict serious injury, perhaps death, on others. The deceased's family may be at particular risk. This was an appalling crime, almost beyond contemplation in a civilised society.'

Katherine Knight's papers were marked 'Never to be released'.

At the Mulawa Women's Correctional Centre (now known as Silverwater Women's Correctional Centre), she initially worked as a cleaner in the governor's office, but now works in a headphone factory.

It has been 19 years since she was taken into custody, now a white-haired 63-year-old woman with a benign smile, with twinkling eyes behind owlish glasses. Knight has apparently found religion, paints, knits, makes pottery and is known as 'The Nanna' by other inmates. However, prison officers wisely never take their eyes off her and it is said that she can't have a cellmate in case she kills again.

And, despite her alleged culinary skills, she is not, unsurprisingly, allowed near the kitchen – and knives!

Sex, Drugs and the Death of a Businessman

'An over-indulgence of anything, even something as
pure as water, can intoxicate.'
– Criss Jami, *Venus in Arms*

David Monlun was a wealthy French-born businessman. He moved to Sydney with his ex-wife in 1996 and went on to establish a couple of successful businesses: Repworld, a transport agency, and Bistrow, an online wine company. During that time, he met an attractive young woman, Sarah Manning, who was 10 years his junior, and in 2003 they had a daughter. That was followed in 2004 by a wedding in Hawaii, although Monlun claimed he'd only gone ahead with the ceremony to appease his girlfriend.

Monlun's success made him wealthy and enabled him to live a lifestyle that we mere mortals can only fantasise about. He displayed all the visible trappings of success, such as frequent travel, expensive cars and a luxurious apartment on the harbour.

To the outsider looking in, Monlun had the ideal life, and perhaps it was at one point, but the relationship between him and his wife was volatile and unstable, being fuelled by a deadly mixture of high–octane sex and the regular use of drugs, in particular GHB ('Liquid Fantasy'), which he kept in a large quantity (about 2 litres) in a safe in his bedroom, along with personal papers.

The couple separated in 2005 but maintained a strange relationship that also included Sarah Manning's former boyfriend, Matthew Haar. In 2006, that culminated in Haar kidnapping Monlun at knifepoint and forcing him to take cocaine, although the motive behind that action was never established. A fortnight later, Monlun was lured to Sarah's Randwick apartment, where he was tied up and beaten before being forced by Haar, Manning and another woman to sign over property, including a Harley-Davidson motorcycle. The trio were charged with various assault and kidnapping offences, which saw Haar jailed for a maximum of three years and three months and the other accomplices given three–year good-behaviour bonds. Despite all that, Monlun and Manning reunited five years later and on 29 May 2011 the two of them, together with Jamie Philip, a GHB user, held a drug-filled party at Monlun's luxurious penthouse apartment overlooking Darling Harbour. Their drugs of choice were GHB and ice (methylamphetamine). The session lasted until just before 3.20 am, and shortly after, Monlun bid his guests farewell and staggered off to bed.

In the early hours of the following morning, he was found lying face down on his bed by his seven-year-old daughter. He was cold to the touch and wearing a blue polo T-shirt, a grey jumper and striped pyjamas. Alarmed that she couldn't wake her father, his daughter contacted her 14-year-old half-sister, who was at school.

An ambulance was promptly called, and the ambulance officers carried out a number of routine medical tests, including checking Monlun's pulse, but they were far too late, the 40-year-old was already dead. His body was later taken to the Glebe Department of Forensic Medicine to determine the cause of his death.

The post-mortem was carried out by Dr Andrew Colebatch at 9.30 am the day after. The examination revealed a number of minor abrasions on Monlun's body, as well as fluid accumulation in his lungs and airways thick with mucoid secretion, typical symptoms of an overdose of a central nervous system depressant. That was borne out by the subsequent toxicology report, which revealed that a blood sample taken at the post-mortem was found to contain gamma-hydroxybutyrate (GHB) 240 milligrams per litre, methylamphetamine 0.45 milligrams per litre and amphetamine 0.04 milligrams per litre. I concluded that the level of GHB detected in Mr David Monlun's blood was consistent with an overdosage of the drug. I was also of the opinion that the blood concentration of GHB, together with an elevated level of methylamphetamine, would have led to his death.

An inquest into the circumstances surrounding Monlun's death was held before the deputy state coroner, Ms Sharon Freund, on 15 July 2013. The inquest was told that during the evening of 29 May 2011 and the early morning of 30 May, Sarah Manning and Jamie Philip had been in Monlun's apartment, and in his opening address, Mr Simon Buchen, the council assisting the coroner, said they had been the last people to see Monlun alive. He then stated that the inquest would examine their behaviour prior to his death, as well as how the businessman came to consume his fatal overdose of GHB.

He also told the court that a few hours prior to his death, Monlun had bought return plane tickets to New Zealand for himself and his daughter over the internet, commenting, 'This circumstance, together with other evidence, would appear to be inconsistent with suicide. He [Mr Monlun] enjoyed a good standard of living and visible trappings of success, such as expensive cars, frequent travel and a sizeable apartment.'

Turning to the relationship between Monlun and Sarah Manning, he said it had been volatile and had displayed 'obsessive conduct'. He continued by saying, 'The consumption of ice and GHB, and drug-fuelled sexual encounters appear to have been a significant feature of the relationship.'

CCTV from inside the apartment showed David Monlun, Sarah Manning and Jamie Philip taking what appeared to be GHB together. Further footage showed Sarah Manning leaving the apartment at various times before returning, and after she and Jamie Philip had left, Monlun becoming unsteady on his feet and dropping a phone.

His Repworld business associate, Raymond Harrison, said that Sarah Manning could 'smell money' and was a 'poisonous woman' who'd inquired about Monlun's will only days after he died. 'She rang and said David had said to her on the event of his death that she should ring me and I would fix everything.' He further said Sarah Manning had also called their business associate, Nicholas Papaix. 'It was both the opinion of Nicholas and mine, Sarah was seeking an alibi regarding her involvement or contact with David and his death.' Harrison said Mr Monlun had been a good businessman, further commenting, 'David was a loveable rogue. You could never stay angry with him. He was fundamentally a good person who I think lost his way near the end of his life. He was a good family man. All of his employees were absolutely loyal and still love him to this day.'

When asked how he felt at the time, Harrison replied, 'I was angry. I blame Sarah for what happened to David.'

The inquest also heard from other witnesses, who described Monlun and Sarah Manning's volatile drug-fuelled relationship, together with the extortion kidnappings involving Matthew Haar. David Monlun's mother, Irene, read out a victim–impact statement, in which she described her son as a 'loveable joker and a good son,' further saying, 'David, as every human being, had his imperfections.'

With time running short and further police enquiries to be made, the court was adjourned until August 2014, and then again until July 2015. The subsequent inquest revealed how David Monlun had resumed his relationship with Sarah Manning despite their previous difficulties, which had intensified in the weeks leading up to his death.

CCTV footage showed that on the night of his death, he and Sarah Manning were partying with several friends and family associates, including Sarah's mother, Jennifer, and Jamie Philip. Sarah Manning and Jamie Philip were seen leaving Monlun's apartment around 4 am with a number of shopping bags.

The coroner ruled out the possibility that David Monlun had deliberately taken his own life and determined that he had either accidentally overdosed or that '… the drugs were deliberately administered to Mr Monlun by another person.' She further noted that photographs on Monlun's mobile, taken three days before his death, showed Sarah Manning posing with a very large amount of cash. 'Such large sums of money and drugs could provide strong motivations to persons to administer a substance, so that the theft could be administered. The persons of interest all have interwoven lives fuelled by deception, sex and illicit drugs. All have reasons to lie and protect themselves.'

She found that Sarah Manning and Jamie Philip remained persons of interest in relation to the death of David Monlun and referred the matter back to the Unsolved Homicide Squad for further investigation.

Readers are encouraged to call Crime Stoppers on 1800 333 000 with any information that may assist investigators to conclude this matter.

A Dog and a Dame in a Ditch: Who Murdered Maureen McLaughlin?

'The darkness of the soul is not lighted by
moving the body to another place.'
– Eastern proverb

Mrs Wanda Steele was an avid bushwalker. Whenever the weather was suitable, she liked nothing better than a hike through some mountainous area or other. And so it was on 13 April 1992 when she set out looking for some bottlebrush and lilac blooms. Shortly before midday, she made her way along the State Mine Gully Road, a thoroughfare adjacent to the Blue Mountains National Park, enjoying her surroundings and the freedom of the wide-open space. As she walked, she saw something protruding out of the ground, a little way in the distance. She didn't think any more about it until she drew level, when what she saw almost made her heave. It was a human arm and hand; the skin, infested with blowflies, peeling away from the flesh and bone. After taking a few minutes to recover her sensibilities, she immediately contacted the Lithgow police, who were soon on the scene.

Lithgow is a small town situated in the Central Tablelands of New

South Wales. It was once a thriving coal mining area, but its glory days are well behind it, most people now recognising the place as an historical tourist destination. A two-hour drive west of Sydney, it nestles among several national parks, one of which is the Blue Mountains National Park.

★

The spot where Mrs Steele made her gruesome discovery was a favourite night-time parking haunt for local young people who cared little for the natural beauty of the area, despoiling it with all kinds of associated trash such as empty drink cans, used condoms, pieces of foil and even bongs.

The police team quickly donned protective clothing and secured the site before beginning the onerous task of clearing the debris that was lying on and around the immediate vicinity of the arm and hand. Having removed the rubbish, they started excavating the coarse river sand and stones that surrounded the protruding limb, proceeding slowly and carefully, as they were not sure whether the arm and hand were all there was or if they would find more body parts.

It wasn't, however, a straightforward operation, as they started uncovering all kinds of scrap and detritus. Amongst the many finds were pieces of corrugated iron; a blue, 20-litre drum; a used automobile engine oil filter, Ryco Z37 brand; an empty, clear plastic, soft-drink bottle; four pieces of white PVC insulating tape; an empty, woven plastic sack, marked 'Pigeon Feed'; and a blue, floral patterned, ladies bolero, containing a bunch of keys in the left pocket and a brooch, in the shape of a marijuana leaf, attached to the front right.

The operation took quite some time, but they eventually accessed a body in its shallow grave. A cursory look revealed it to be that of an adult female. She was naked from the shoulders down, save for a white brassiere and a red and white skivvy. Her bra was fastened at the back and had been pulled up at the front, exposing her breasts. Further inspection showed a number of rings on the right hand and three earrings in the right ear lobe, with a further earring under the left ear. At first glance, the head appeared to be resting on a piece of coarse carpet, but after the body had been lifted, it was found to be the rotting carcass of a dog, which when moved, revealed two .22 calibre cartridges, both of them spent.

By the time the body had been recovered, photographs taken and exhibits meticulously detailed, night was falling, so the Lithgow Volunteer Rescue Association set up floodlighting so the work could continue. Shortly afterwards, Dr K. Fields, the government medical officer for the Lithgow district, arrived at the crime scene and examined the body, which was then transported to the Lithgow mortuary, where it was washed and examined externally by Dr Fields himself.

The most striking thing about the corpse was that it was decorated with numerous tattoos. Dr Fields duly photographed and recorded each one. There was an eight-point star on the inside left ankle, a rose with two faces on the left thigh, a marijuana leaf on the left buttock with the words 'Life be out of it', an angel on the right buttock, a stylised vulture sitting on a post with the words 'DEAD END 666' on the left upper arm, the word 'ARIES' and its symbol, along with the words 'Alice Cooper' with the symbol of a mouth and tongue on the right thigh, and tattoos of hinges on both inner elbows.

She had clearly been a young woman with attitude.

Finally, a set of fingerprints was taken for identification purposes before the body was encased in a body bag, which was then fastened and placed into a sealed refrigerator to await its final trip to the Sydney City Mortuary, in Glebe, the following morning.

The body was identified as that of Maureen Ann McLaughlin, but the presence of the dead dog and the two spent .22 calibre cartridges were a real puzzler. What was their significance to Ms McLaughlin's death?

The dog was identified as a Rottweiler-kelpie cross and traced to its owner, Ceanne Gwendoline Towers. The case detectives were dispatched to interview her, discovering that Ceanne had been in a long-term relationship with a woodchopper, Graham 'Chook' Fowler, who allegedly dealt cannabis to supplement his income. The couple had two children and Sheba, the Rottweiler-kelpie.

Further enquiries showed that Fowler was a man with a history of violence, and he'd often engaged in both physical and mental aggression against Ceanne. On one occasion, during a domestic argument, he'd armed himself with a kitchen knife and tried to stab her, but the knife had struck the kitchen table and deflected into his wrist.

He'd also been violent to his ex-wife, and there was a story going round that he'd once thrown a woman from his car while it was still moving, causing serious injuries. Like many people, his aggressive attitude intensified after he'd been drinking.

The incident that led to the death of Ceanne's Rottweiler-kelpie occurred after Fowler flipped out over the dog digging holes in the rear yard of their home. On 14 December 1991, he took a .22 calibre semi-automatic rifle out of a cupboard, put the dog into a utility and drove to Newnes Drift (State Mine Gully), an area he knew well from his work, and killed it with two shots to the head.

Meanwhile, Ceanne had rung the Lithgow Police, fearing for the dog's safety, but she was too late. Fowler returned home and admitted to what he'd done, whereupon a distressed and tearful Ceanne contacted her mother and father, telling them what had happened. The three of them went to search Newnes Drift and found Sheba's body. Ceanne's father then took a pick and shovel out of his vehicle and dug a deep grave in which to place the body. When they finished the burial, Ceanne marked the site with a pink-beaded, white plastic cross.

At the same time as the police were chasing up the possible dog connection, the post-mortem into Maureen McLaughlin took place. The morning after her body had been discovered, it was collected from the Lithgow mortuary and driven to the Glebe Department of Forensic Medicine, in Sydney, where it was formally identified by its fingerprints and Maureen's distraught parents.

The post-mortem, carried out by forensic pathologist Dr Lillian Schwartz, revealed a number of injuries to Maureen's body, and a sample of maggots (*Calliphora stygia larvae*) was taken to be analysed in order to provide an estimate of the time of death, but unfortunately, owing to a snafu before arrival at the laboratory, it wasn't possible. In addition, a number of swabs, smears and specimens were collected and delivered to the Department of Forensic Medicine.

Dr Schwartz concluded that although the decompositional changes of the deceased suggested a period of approximately 7 to 14 days after death and some of the injuries seen on the body might have been caused after death, the large number of head injuries and bruises seen on the body strongly suggested that Maureen had died as a result of the head injuries.

An analysis of body tissues (taken because a suitable blood sample was not available) revealed that there was nordiazapam 0.42 milligram per kilogram present in Maureen's liver and 0.01 milligram per kilogram of the same substance in her stomach. I concluded that at those levels the drug was not responsible for her death, and although the spleen and muscle samples contained small amounts of alcohol, that was most likely due to the fermentation of glucose in the body from bacterial and/or yeasts during decomposition.

A later post-mortem confirmed the findings of Dr Schwartz that the evidence of head trauma and possible strangulation indicators were the probable causes contributing to Maureen's death.

And so it was on to the inquest to determine the circumstances surrounding it.

It took place on 6 July 1993, at Lithgow Coroner's Court, before the Coroner, Mr Derek Hand.

Members of Maureen's family and some acquaintances came forward in an effort to shed some light on the matter, but other than evidence that she'd been a heavy smoker and that, unusually for her, she'd left her cigarettes in her flat on the night of her disappearance, scant progress was made towards solving the mystery, and after two days, the court was unable to reach any sort of conclusion. However, the coroner did comment on the coincidence of Graham Fowler shooting his de facto's dog and the fact that Maureen's body had been found where the dog had been buried. He was, though, quite satisfied that was all it was, and that there was nothing to connect Fowler and Ceanne with Maureen, and that it was all just an extreme coincidence.

Unable to determine either the manner or cause of Maureen's death, the coroner returned an open verdict, meaning the case remained open, but with no nominated person of interest.

A reward of $100,000 was offered for information, but met with no response, so when the Western Region Unsolved Homicide Team renewed its investigation into the case, designating it Strike Force Checkley, in September 2009, it was increased to $200,000. At the time of writing this story, the reward money is still available, so if you have any information that may help investigators to close this cold case and bring the perpetrator(s) to justice, please call Crime Stoppers on 1800 333 000.

Death by Herbal Tea

'Good medicine [often] tastes bitter.'
– Chinese Proverb

Accidental or deliberate consumption of poisonous herbs has become an increasingly common problem over the last few years in Australia. This is no doubt due to an increased interest in alternative medicine, using herbal preparations, and in particular, traditional Chinese medicine (TCM), which is favoured by Asian immigrants who may be wary of Western medicine and be seeking a more traditional treatment.

TCM relies on complex herbal preparations as well as minerals and animal parts to treat a variety of ailments. However, adverse effects have been reported, many of them from misuse or abuse of Chinese medicine. Some herbs have a narrow therapeutic range, where the difference between a therapeutic dose and a toxic dose is very close, and so great care needs to be exercised to ensure the right quantity is prescribed and dispensed. Herbs such as Chinese monkshood (*Aconitum carmichaelii*) and the *Aconitum* species in general have narrow therapeutic ranges, leading to toxic effects being frequently reported. However, the herb has retained its place as an effective medicinal treatment in TCM for a number of conditions, including yang deficiency (general debility), severe pain, decreased kidney function, cardiac weakness and gastric pain.

Unfortunately, herbal remedies are not subject to the rigorous quality control measures that regular pharmaceutical medicines have to undergo in order to be registered, manufactured, prescribed and dispensed, and that has led to some very unfortunate outcomes as this case illustrates.

On 13 May 2013, Mr Xing Min Lee attended a clinic run by Dr Xiang Dong to seek treatment for his psoriasis, which may have been related to his arthritic condition. Dr Dong, being a traditional Chinese doctor, gave him a mixture of herbs widely used in the Chinese community, which Mr Lee consumed in the form of a tea (the dried herbs being infused in hot water) prepared by his wife, Shaofen Lee, who was au fait with the techniques needed to prepare the traditional medicinal tea. After taking the herbal mixture, Mr Lee told her that he believed his psoriasis rashes were improving, but his back pain had got worse. (The latter problem was more likely due to his work as a forklift driver at the Flemington Markets and the physical nature of some of his duties, which involved a certain amount of lifting.)

Eight days later, on 21 May, during the morning, Mr Lee undertook a routine blood test for his diabetes mellitus condition and then returned home, where he contacted his wife, who was at work, to ask for instructions on how to make the herbal tea.

A few hours later, around 2 pm, Mrs Lee returned home to find vomit on the lounge-room floor. It looked like phlegm and the Chinese medicine components. Alarmed, she ran upstairs and found her husband asleep in bed. He woke up and said, 'I'm very hungry. I don't feel well. Can you cook me some congee [a type of rice porridge] to eat? And don't trouble me, I'm very tired.'

Mrs Lee dutifully went down stairs, cleared up the vomit and prepared some congee for her distressed husband. While she was busy in the kitchen, she heard what sounded like someone falling over. She rushed upstairs to find her husband on the bathroom floor, gasping for air.

'What? What? What?' was all she could say on seeing the distressing sight of her husband's situation. Still gasping, Mr Lee indicated he needed the toilet, so she helped him up from the floor and placed him on the seat.

'I can't do it,' Mr Lee complained. 'My back is excruciating. The pain is like nerves are being pulled.'

Mrs Lee thought some Chinese medical oil might help and rubbed some onto his back, but her husband's condition didn't improve.

'It feels like my insides are cramping. It's very painful, very painful.'

As Mrs Lee applied more oil, she called out to her sister, Amy Zong, who was visiting at the time, 'Please call the ambulance straight away. He's suffering.'

It was approximately 2.50 pm.

In the meantime, Mr Lee's condition continued to worsen. He began to scream in pain and struggle to breathe. Just as the ambulance officers arrived and ran upstairs, he stopped moaning and moving. The officers promptly commenced CPR, but he didn't respond, so after about 30 minutes, they decided to get him to Auburn Hospital as quickly as possible.

After an anxious wait, a doctor and two nurses approached the family, and told them the sad news – Mr Lee had passed away.

A crime scene was subsequently set up and a quantity of herbs from the Lees' garage was collected and labelled. Forensic police also took a sample of the soaked herbs from the pot containing the herbal mixture that Mr Lee had brewed. Those specimens were packaged, labelled and logged before being dispatched to the Southern Cross University, Plant Science, and Analytical Research Laboratory (ARL) for botanical examination and chemical analysis.

Initially, the herbal mixture was forwarded to a Chinese herbalist and acupuncturist for comment on the herbal mix content, but it wasn't considered unusual in any way. However, two herbal species that aren't scheduled for use by Chinese herbalists by the Therapeutic Goods Administration (TGA) in Australia were identified in the concoction, namely *Aconitum carmichaelii* and *Typhonium giganteu*. Consequently, the laboratory looked for the presence of aconitine, a highly toxic alkaloid present in one of the Chinese herbs (*Aconitum carmichaelii*), also known as fuzi, but the analysis carried out on the submitted test samples of herbal tea residues prepared from the herbal mixture found no detectable traces of the alkaloid.

A bag of dried Chinese herbs used to prepare the tea was also botanically examined, in particular looking for plant material consistent with fuzi. It was found that the herbal mixture was consistent with 12 different plant sources. Of those, two contained the botanical characteristics of fuzi. Further examination identified one of the herbs as the lateral roots of *Aconitum carmichaelii* (fuzi) and the other as the rhizome of *Typhonium giganteum*, known in Chinese medicine as *zhi baifu zi*.

Further chemical analysis showed that while the herbal material didn't contain free aconitine, it did contain the monoesters of aconitine, which, according to the *Chinese Pharmacopoeia*, are supposedly produced when the raw material is processed and reduce the toxicity of the material so that it can be effective as a medicine.

The human liver contains many ways to detox the various substances that we consume, be they in food or medicines, and various drugs in ester form are readily de-esterified in the liver, releasing the free drug and/or toxin produced into the bloodstream. That may get rid of the toxin from the body or make it worse through the creation of a more poisonous substance brought about by metabolic change.

The *Typhonium* sp. in the mixture presented something of a mystery, but a number of chemicals in high concentrations that were lipophilic (fat soluble), with a number of significant toxic components, appeared, and the *Chinese Pharmacopoeia* warns, 'Be cautions [sic] when the unprocessed tuber is taken orally.'

It was clear that a special preparation procedure was needed to render the herbal tea beneficial and not toxic, which is the problem with herbal medications. An almost ritual procedure needs to be followed to turn potentially complex poisonous mixtures into a medicinal tea. Unfortunately, Mr Lee appeared to be unaware of that.

For his particular preparation, it was necessary to cook the herbs for a certain period before adding five bowls of water, which were then boiled down to one. It was a procedure Mr Lee's wife had carried out before, but on that fateful day, a crucial step in the preparation of the herbal brew had been missing, resulting in a toxic tea instead of a medicinal one.

Mr Lee's body arrived at the Glebe Department of Forensic Medicine on the morning of 22 May 2013. A post-mortem was carried out at 9 am the following day.

At the examination, evidence of medical intervention (ECG pads, resuscitation pads, laryngeal mask, and infusion solution) was observed. There were 'multifocal skin lesions, (psoriasiform); pulmonary congestion … and oedema; moderate fatty changes, macrovesicular, liver; steatohepatitis, liver' and curiously, the stomach contained '500 ml of tan liquid and rare leaf-like material (herbal tea leaves?).'

A subsequent toxicology report of a blood sample taken at the time was found to only contain metformin 1.0 milligrams per litre. No alcohol or other drugs were detected.

Metformin is an oral hypoglycaemic agent for the treatment of maturity-onset diabetes. It's available under several trade names including Diabex. Its therapeutic range is between 1 and four milligrams per litre. The level of metformin detected in Mr Lee's blood was within that, indicating a moderate ingestion of the drug.

I subsequently concluded that the symptoms displayed by Mr Xing Lee before his death appeared consistent with aconite poisoning. However, an examination of his stomach contents (which contained 'rare leaf-like material') may have confirmed this finding.

The stomach contents sample was sent off to ESR laboratories in New Zealand for further testing to determine the presence of aconitine and related substances. Surprisingly, the result came back negative. This poison was certainly elusive.

Unfortunately, the liver sample – the next tissue of choice after blood – was not available, so it was time to test his urine sample.

Aconitine is one of number of highly poisonous alkaloids present in the toxic plant genus *Aconitum*. A number of *Aconitum* species contain significant amounts of aconitine and related alkaloids. The alkaloid is present in the leaves, stem and root of *Aconitum* sp. The toxic aconite plants include various species such as *Aconitum napellus*, which is more commonly known as monkshood or wolfsbane, and *Aconitum carmichaelii*, better known as Chinese aconite or Chinese wolfsbane. Toxins extracted from the plants were traditionally used to kill wolves, hence the name 'wolf's bane'. However, most of the 250 or so species are very poisonous and must be handled with care.

Chinese wolfsbane has been used in Chinese herbal medicine for treatment of a variety of ailments, including skin diseases, rheumatism, arthritis, cold hands and feet, deficiency in kidneys, body aches and all 'yang injuries'. The usual dosage is between 3 and 8 grams. However, the fresh drug is very poisonous, although it becomes somewhat less toxic after drying. Nevertheless, it should be brewed for a long time.

The alkaloid generally held responsible for the plant's toxic properties is aconitine, although the less potent hypaconitine, jesaconitine and mesaconitine are also poisonous.

Various toxic symptoms due to aconite ingestion include nausea, vomiting, numbness and palsy of the extremities. Other symptoms include diarrhoea, difficulty in breathing and cardiac arrhythmia. Death may occur from paralysis of the heart or the respiratory centre.

Aconitine has been known as the 'Queen of Poisons' and has featured in a number of notable deaths throughout history, including George Henry Lamson who used the poison to dispose of a relative. He was a doctor, and he went from being a decorated war hero who served with distinction during the wars that ravaged Europe and the Balkans to being a bankrupt drug addict and murderer. During the war in Romania and Serbia, he served his time as a surgeon, returning to England, where he practised in Bournemouth. Unfortunately, he became addicted to morphine, and that addiction drained his finances so badly that he became desperate for money.

It was then that he decided to use the Queen of Poisons to murder his disabled 18-year-old brother-in-law, Percy Malcolm, for an inheritance of 3000 pounds, a princely sum in those days. He visited Percy at his boarding school and gave him a slice of Dundee cake, along with a capsule that was later tested and found to contain aconitine. He was eventually arrested and tried in March 1882 at the Old Bailey and found guilty of murder. The following month, he was hanged in Wandsworth Prison.

Another death attributable to aconitine poisoning was that of 25-year-old Canadian actor, Andre Noble, who died on 30 July 2004 when he apparently mistook a monkshood for an edible flower during a hiking trip with his aunt on Fair Island, Newfoundland. He became very ill at her cabin near Centreville, Indian Bay, and later died while being conveyed to hospital.

More recently, in 2009, another notorious aconitine poisoning occurred. Dubbed by the media as the Curry Killer case, it centred on Lakhvir Kaur Singh, aged 45, and her former lover of 16 years, Lakhvinder Cheema, aged 39. Desperate to prevent their forthcoming marriage on Valentine's Day, Singh broke into the house in Feltham, Middlesex that Lakhvinder Cheema shared with his fiancée, Gurjeet Choongh, aged 21, and spiked a prepared chicken curry in the fridge with Indian aconite (*Aconitium ferox*).

When the couple returned home, they settled down for their evening meal, unaware the food had been poisoned. Lakhvinder (also ironically known as Lucky) was very hungry and tucked into a second helping. Fortunately, his fiancée only had a small portion. Within minutes, the couple experienced the toxic effects of the poison. Before Lakhvinder fell unconscious, he said he suspected Lakhvir Singh of the foul deed because an attempt on his life had been made some time earlier. He was taken to hospital, but died soon after. Gurjeet Choongh was placed in a medically induced coma and survived.

Lakhvir Singh was arrested and tried on 11 February 2010 at the Old Bailey, where she was found guilty of murder. She was sentenced to life imprisonment with a minimum term of 23 years.

★

The inquest into Xing Min Lee's death found that he'd been a popular, much loved and hard-working man, and his death had been caused by misadventure. In other words, it had been accidental.

Many cases of poisoning have resulted from poor quality prescription practice, dispensary error, and the use of a greater than the recommended dose or inadequate boiling of processed aconite roots during herbal tea preparation. Given that Mr Lee had consumed the same herbal mixture previously, which had been prepared by his wife, it appears that the most likely scenario was one of inadequate preparation of the decoction, probably through insufficient boiling of the herbal mixture.

Sadly, the herbal tea that was supposed to take away his arthritic pain, instead took his life.

An Evening with Mr Buggers

'Abuse is never deserved, it is an exploitation of
innocence and physical disadvantage,
which is perceived as an opportunity by the abuser.'
– *Lorraine Nilon,* **Breaking Free from the Chains of Silence**

Nitrous oxide has been used in dentistry and medicine for over 150 years. Discovered in 1776 by Joseph Priestly, its potential as an anaesthetic was only recognised 23 years later by Humphrey Davy, and it didn't come into general usage until after 1860. Non-flammable and nearly odourless, with a slight sweetish smell, it's a good analgesic, but won't produce complete anaesthesia at safe concentrations (65% oxygen) and so is used mainly as an analgesic (pain relieving) agent in dentistry. It's relatively insoluble in body tissues and fluids and so induction and recovery are generally quite rapid.

It gained its other moniker of 'laughing gas' because of its effects before anaesthesia, when it produces a type of laugh along with a feeling of euphoria. As a result, it was (and still is) used recreationally at parties in much the same way that ecstasy is used at rave parties today. The substance can readily be obtained from medical supplies or whipped cream cans, where it's used as a propellant that mixes in the liquid cream. When the cream escapes from the can, the gas expands and in the process whips the cream into a foam. However, it isn't all fun and games, as the inhalation of 40% nitrous oxide in air causes confusion and sedation, while a level of 80% causes unconsciousness in most people.

*

In 2000, Dee Why, a coastal suburb of northern Sydney, in common with many other towns throughout the country, had a church youth group where the young people of the community could socialise in an apparently caring religious setting, watching videos and playing Xbox and other games. Good fun was had by all every Friday night.

One of the youth leaders, a Mr Buggers (not his real name, but one that was deemed to be very apt at the time) took a special interest in the teenage boys in his care, and invited a few of them to his residence on a warm Saturday in August. One of those was 15-year-old Scott Evers, who was looking forward to spending some more time with his friends in a relaxed environment. He arrived at midday and knocked on the door. Mr Buggers parted the drawn curtains and peered out. Seeing Scott, he smiled and went to open the door, welcoming the boy inside. Two of Scott's friends were already there, but to Scott's horror, they were in various states of consciousness and neither was wearing any clothing from the waist down. Scott turned round and left, ignoring Mr Buggers' attempts (both verbal and physical) to get him to stay, and reported what he'd seen to his parents, who went to the police.

The police acted swiftly and interviewed Mr Buggers and his victims, in the process uncovering a whole series of sexual abuses and Mr Buggers' modus operandi. As a local school teacher and church elder, he'd gained a position of trust and authority within the community, which, up until Scott, had deterred his victims from outing him. Being youngsters, they thought that they wouldn't be believed and would possibly even be punished for making up stories. Added to that, Mr Buggers also used his position to make credible threats of what might happen to them if they were to tell.

Mr Buggers ran what he called his 'creaming club', which he set up in order to entice young men, ranging from the ages of 11 to 23, into being sexual participants. He'd use his many wiles to attract bored or otherwise unemployed males to his home, where he'd administer them doses of nitrous oxide via various whipped cream canisters which had had the cream removed and replaced by nitrous oxide gas bulbs. The young men, promised that it was just a bit of fun, then inhaled the gas. After a brief period of 'laughter', they became semi-conscious, experiencing varying degrees of disinhibition. Unaware of what was going on, or even where they were, they were then sexually abused by Mr Buggers.

Mr Buggers was subsequently charged with a number of offences relating to sexual/indecent assaults upon young male persons under section 38 of the Crimes Act in that he 'did unlawfully cause to be taken chloroform or stupefying drug or thing to commit an indictable offence'.

One of his victims testified that he'd done it to a whole range of people and had photos of them on his computer, while another said that he'd passed out and when he'd woken up, Buggers had been feeling his private parts. When asked how he felt when he woke up to find Buggers putting his mouth over his penis, he replied, 'I don't know. I felt like I was stoned.' Interviews with other victims were disturbingly similar, with one saying that Buggers had pretty much raped him.

I was asked if I could say, in my expert opinion, that nitrous oxide was a stupefying drug or thing, and was disinhibiting or un-inhibiting to the user, which I could and did, as did the other experts who were called.

The case may have been about laughing gas, but the judge and jury were anything but amused.

Mr Buggers was sentenced to 13 years imprisonment with a non-parole period of nine and a half years, giving him plenty of time to reflect on his former lifestyle and make appropriate amendments. But can a leopard change its spots? Only time will tell.

Tulips for Holly:
Death of a 'Wild Child'

'My candle burns at both ends. It will not last the night;
But ah, my foes, and oh, my friends –
it gives a lovely light'
– Edna St Vincent Millay

Holly Violet Francis-Burroughs was a Canadian expatriate. She was a real party girl who loved socialising and chilling out with friends. Her family background was somewhat unconventional to say the least; her father was allegedly the financial head of an outlaw motorcycle gang in Canada, and when she was born, her mother was a crack cocaine addict. Holly, her brother and two sisters were abandoned by their mother when they were very young, having no contact since then.

At the age of 16, she migrated to Australia with her aunt, her younger brother, Ray, and her sister, Bonny Francis-Carroll, and they set up home in the Sydney suburb of Narraweena. Later on, she met up with a local young man, and shortly after, they moved into an apartment together, in Manly. A couple of years after that, Holly's aunt returned to Canada with Bonny. Ray followed a year later. Holly and her young man stayed in the Manly apartment for two years before taking up residence in a humble housing commission bedsitter with a kitchen and bathroom at Dora Street, North Ryde, Sydney.

The unit was a short distance from a popular watering hole, the Ranch Hotel (formerly known as El Rancho). Located in Marsfield, an area bordered by suburbs, including North Ryde, Macquarie Park, Eastwood and Epping, it boasts three-and-a-half-star accommodation, which is popular with Macquarie Business Park guests, local tradesmen and professionals, and people visiting Macquarie University, Macquarie Hospital and Curzon Hall. Holly frequently met up with friends for drinks and a chat there, but some of those friends were less than desirable, offering her drugs in return for sexual favours.

With her colourful background, it wasn't too surprising that she was a bit of a wild child. Unfortunately, she also loved 'ice' (a potent form of methylamphetamine), ecstasy (MDMA), amphetamine and any other stimulant that would bring her up. She was one for burning the candle at both ends and enjoyed high-risk sex in public places with a number of different men, one of whom was special to her – Dahkota Salcedo. However, he had a lengthy police record. A bad boy, noted for violence against women, along with robbery and property offences, including breaking and entering, he had a string of offences as long as your arm. Holly even said to a close friend after an argument, 'I got in the middle of it and Dahkota choked me until I was unconscious.'

He was a poor choice, but Holly was apparently in love with him. She was 'the moth to his flame'. Salcedo, who was in his twenties, was about six foot (1.83 metres), a Pacific Islander, good looking with dark eyes and dark hair. He also lived in a housing commission area, dubbed for some odd reason, 'Smurfs Village'.

However, a tragic tale was about to unfold.

Thursday, 7 June 2012 was cold and breezy. At about 9.20 am Adam Stenberg, who lived in the same unit complex as Holly, dropped by her flat to collect the $25 owed to him. It was his third attempt to contact her that day, having previously tried at 7.30 am and 8.30 am. He'd been a little concerned at the lack of response and so decided to make a personal visit.

After knocking on Holly's door for some time, again receiving no indication that she was there, he gave the door a gentle push. It swung open with ease and he could see signs of a previous forced entry. Upon entering the unit, he saw Holly. She was fully clothed in winter attire, with track pants and a pair of laced up running shoes. A scarf was wrapped loosely around her neck and she appeared to be dozing on the bed. Adam walked over to her and immediately twigged that something wasn't quite right. She was lying in an awkward position and her eyes were half shut. She was very still and he was unable arouse her. At that point, Adam realised she was probably dead, so he immediately contacted her close neighbours, Steven Marchant, Patricia Mitchell and Anthony Cowan, who came round to Holly's unit while Adam checked for vital signs. Unfortunately, there were none, so a 000 call was made to alert the emergency services.

An ambulance arrived at just gone 9.30 am and the officers carried out a basic examination of Holly's body, confirming that she'd died and was showing signs of rigor mortis. At about the same time, the police also appeared, and they made visual inspections, noting some unusual marks on her neck. Crime scene officers took photographs of her body and collected various exhibits.

Dr Matthew Orde, an on-call pathologist, arrived at about 3 pm and examined her body. He noted the extensive petechial haemorrhages on her face and neck and formed the opinion that Holly had been strangled. Holly was known as a chronic prescription medication abuser, together with various other illicit drugs such as ice, ecstasy and cannabis, and whether she'd been strangled or suffered from an overdose, it appeared that her wild life had caught up with her.

Her body was taken to the Glebe Department of Forensic Medicine that afternoon, and the post-mortem was carried out by Dr Matthew Orde at 9.15 am the following morning. He observed a number of injuries, some being minor scars due to earlier feeble attempts at self-harm. But most notably, 'There was moderately intense congestion of the face and under surface of the chin. In this region there were numerous petechial and larger frank cutaneous haemorrhages. Corresponding dense petechial haemorrhages were noted over the scleral aspects of the left and right eyes and within the conjunctival recesses of the upper and lower eyelids of both eyes. There was also a dense shower of petechial haemorrhages within the inner aspects of the lips and over the external aspects of the gums.' Additionally, 'there were prominent congestive features to the face, with numerous facial and conjunctival petechial haemorrhages, and with a neat linear lower cut-off over the neck.'

In other words, it appeared Holly had died through strangulation. A petechial haemorrhage is a small pinpoint red mark that is an indicative sign of asphyxia caused by some external means of obstructing a person's airways. Their presence quite often indicates a death by hanging, smothering or manual strangulation. The haemorrhages result when blood leaks from the tiny capillaries in the eyes, which can rupture due to increased pressure on the veins in the head when the airways are blocked. If petechial haemorrhages and facial congestion are present, there is a strong indication that asphyxia by strangulation was the cause of death. Holly showed both symptoms, and it initially looked like a clear case of murder. Curiously, the hyoid bone and laryngeal cartilages were still intact. If those had been ruptured and/or damaged, they would have provided confirmatory signs of strangulation.

But things in real life are rarely so simple. We humans are complex creatures and expected outcomes may not eventuate. In addition, there was the toxicology report to consider, and that further complicated the case.

Holly's love of drug stimulants was borne out in the report, which showed that a blood sample taken from her body at post-mortem contained amphetamine 2.6 milligrams per litre, methylamphetamine less than 0.02 milligrams per litre, delta-9-tetrahydrocannabinol (THC, the psychoactive component of cannabis) 0.006 milligrams per litre, delta-9-THC acid (the inactive breakdown product of cannabis) 0.021 milligrams per litre, diazepam 0.06 milligrams per litre, nordiazepam 0.19 milligrams per litre, oxazepam 0.04 milligrams per litre, temazepam 0.01 milligrams per litre.

The important player was the elevated level of amphetamine. The others indicated minor drug use, with cannabis and diazepam (Valium), both downers, used to treat the stimulant highs.

I reported that amphetamine (dextroamphetamine, an isomer of amphetamine) is a psychostimulant drug approved for the treatment of attention deficit hyperactivity disorder (ADHD) and narcolepsy. However, methylamphetamine has no approved use in Australia. Both drugs are central nervous system (CNS) stimulants which can impair users' faculties by altering perceptions and judgment and increasing aggressive or risk-taking behaviour during the acute phase of intoxication.

Further, these drugs may also produce hallucinations. Following the stimulation phase, as the blood concentrations of the stimulants decrease, there may be a reactive drug-induced fatigue stage when a user's faculties can be further impaired. During this stage the user may experience drowsiness/sleepiness/fatigue, a slowing of reactions and impairment of perceptions and judgement. After ingestion, both amphetamine and methylamphetamine are rapidly distributed throughout the CNS, where they increase catecholamine activity (and serotonin activity at higher doses), thus producing their psychological effects. Amphetamine has a half-life of 7–4 hours and stays in the user's body for several days depending upon the acidity or alkalinity of their urine.

The blood concentration of methylamphetamine was low indicating either the drug was consumed sometime earlier or that a moderate amount of the drug was ingested. However, the blood concentration of amphetamine is (well) outside the therapeutic range (0.05–0.15 mg/L) and into the lethal range and indicates a very large dosage of the drug was consumed by Ms Francis-Burroughs. Large doses of amphetamine can result in restlessness, anxiety, irritability, hyperactivity and aggressive and/or bizarre behaviour, cerebral vasculitis, myocardial infarction, ischemic stroke and intracranial haemorrhage and have been attributed to abusers of amphetamine/s.

Ms Francis-Burroughs' head and neck showed a number of haemorrhages including petechial and larger frank cutaneous haemorrhages, as recorded in Dr Orde's post-mortem report. Medications such as aspirin or amphetamines may also produce a petechial rash. Dr Orde also notes that, 'The hyoid bone and laryngeal cartilages were intact.' Further, amphetamines can bring about increased sensitivity to stress associated with dopaminergic changes and noradrenergic hyperactivity that may result in stress-related psychiatric disorders.

I concluded, that the blood concentration of amphetamine would have been a contributory factor in Ms Francis-Burroughs' death, by rendering her more susceptible to stress-related psychoactive effects, taking into account her likely high tolerance to the drug (due to her alleged long-term use of dexamphetamine).

This proved to be a controversial finding because many were convinced her death had been caused by murder via strangulation. Sadly, a 'don't-confuse-me-with-the-facts' type attitude seemed to prevail at the time, which made an impartial assessment very difficult. But I was also uncertain, given Holly's background and drug habits.

The toxicology report confirmed that Holly did live life on the edge through her need for stimulants, both chemical and physical, and once done, she needed to 'normalise' her life by taking downers such as cannabis, benzodiazepines (Valium, Serapax, etc.) and Oxycontin (a brand of oxycodone, an opiate pain-reliever). It's a common way of life in the drug subculture, where stimulants are used to go that extra kilometre or improve sexual and/or sporting performance, after which a depressant such as cannabis or drugs such as the benzodiazepines or alcohol are used to reduce the stimulant effects so users can come down and relax and/or sleep.

Unfortunately, Holly would take drugs regardless of how she was feeling. Whether she was sad or happy, it didn't matter, it had become a habit. Every Wednesday (her payday from Centrelink), she'd buy a few grams of cannabis and about 30 tablets of 'Dexy' (dexamphetamine). Occasionally, she would also purchase drugs if someone happened to call by her bedsitter and have drugs for sale. It was said she obtained about 50 Valium tablets and about 15 Oxycontin tablets a week, which she stored in an M&M's mini sweet container and kept on her person at all times, even to the point that she would take it into the bathroom with her. Valium and Oxycontin is a dangerous combination, which if mistakenly taken together, would have ended her life before other events subsequently caught up with her.

Also, every Wednesday, she would regularly take 30 to 40 'Dexy' tablets, and as the drug is an upper, she wouldn't sleep for a few days.

The drug combination/s clearly messed with her brain chemistry, as she was said to be very happy some times and quite depressed at others, at one time making an attempt to take her own life by cutting her left inner forearm with a knife. Her drug use destroyed her life, turning it into a series of uppers and downers.

And then there were the men of dubious reputation in her life, who further complicated matters. Dakhota Salcedo, his brother Brendan, and their friend, Quinn Fillipano. They would go around to her place, stay for a few hours and then leave. As she once said to a close friend, it was, 'same shit, different day'. She would buy food and various people would come to her house and eat it all. As a consequence she lost a lot of weight. Sometimes she would come home and find that her front door had been kicked in and they'd be sitting in her unit watching television and using her facilities. Holly was clearly being taken advantage of, and it appeared the young men wanted more than just friendship. It was a situation fraught with danger.

The tenants in the bedsitter units in Dora Street were a tight-knit community who generally looked out for one another. Holly was very popular and her unit was seen as a drop-in house where friends and acquaintances would often hang out during the day, so it came as an awful surprise that she'd been found dead.

The news was quickly relayed to Holly's friends, who chipped in to present floral tributes, the first being a bunch of tulips. They were followed by many other flowers placed on the fence outside her unit. A sign was also placed on the fence. It read: 'Holly 21 years old found dead in her unit on 7/6/12. Police have found no relatives of poor Holly. May justice be served?'

When police first arrived at the scene on that cold June morning, a day before Holly's twenty-first birthday, it wasn't immediately apparent that her death was suspicious, as there was no weapon, and few clues were found in the house apart from a used condom and satchels containing cannabis residues.

As with many of life's ironies, Holly had apparently been trying to get her life together prior to her death, indicating she was going to stop being a 'tripper junkie bitch'. Prior to that admission, her Facebook page had been filled with references to drugs.

While a number of teary-eyed friends attended her funeral, no family came forward to mourn her loss. A sad end for one so young.

Three months later, after receiving the post-mortem report, the police swung into action and set up Strike Force Arendal to investigate her death because it now appeared she had been murdered, with the preliminary cause of death being due to 'asphyxia due to compression of the neck, as a result of ligature strangulation'.

The vital toxicology report was still some six weeks away.

In the meantime, detectives interviewed many of Holly's friends and associates. But as the investigation continued, one strong suspect began to emerge, and his name was Dakohta Salcedo.

Inquiries revealed that Holly had spent the early part of 6 June 2012 with her friends Patricia Mitchell and Anthony Cowan at their Herring Road unit in Marsfield. During the afternoon, Holly had suggested to her friends that they go to the nearby Ranch Hotel. At about 6.30 pm Dakohta Salcedo had called around to Holly's unit, and while there, they'd had sex. (That activity was denied by Salcedo in an interview five days later with detectives, but later DNA evidence proved overwhelming.) During that time, a storm had affected electrical power to Holly's unit, so an electrician had been called and had set about rectifying the problem. After he'd left, Holly had apparently consumed more pills from her cache and started becoming quite drug affected. At about 1 am on the morning of 7 June, Dakohta Salcedo had fallen asleep, and when he'd woken at about 3 am, he'd found Holly sitting on the floor, propped up against a lounger, giving the impression that she'd overdosed. That scenario seemed to be quite feasible in so far as it went, but didn't answer the question as to why Salcedo hadn't called for medical assistance. Something else was clearly afoot.

Further evidence, painstakingly gathered by detectives, showed that an altercation had occurred between the pair, most likely drug-fuelled, resulting in the fatal outcome.

On 6 March 2013, 25-year-old Dakohta Salcedo was charged with the murder of Holly Violet Francis-Burroughs and appeared at Burwood Local Court.

In September the following year, Salcedo admitted to his mother that he'd pulled Holly's scarf when she'd tried to stop him from leaving her unit, saying, 'She just dropped. I didn't mean it. It was an accident. I didn't mean for her to die.'

Although Salcedo had a poor criminal record (he was on parole at the time of Holly's death and receiving psychiatric treatment for anger management issues toward women), and it looked as if Holly's body had been moved, the fact that the scarf was still in place, together with the level of drugs found in her blood (in particular, amphetamine) made the admission he'd made to his mother appear to be legitimate.

In August 2014, he appeared before Justice Michael Adams at the Supreme Court to answer the charges and for the subsequent sentencing. The earlier murder charge had been withdrawn, but he'd pleaded guilty to, and been convicted of, the lesser charge of manslaughter following a trial earlier that year.

I appeared in court to provide expert evidence and said the stimulant, amphetamine, present in her blood, was the main player (along with a cocktail of other drugs) in the tragic scenario, and that the drug would have increased Holly's sensitivity to stress and episode recurrence. The 'unnecessarily violent' attack by Salcedo on his lover was sufficient to tip her over the edge, resulting in the fatality. Previously, the court had heard that Holly had been addicted to various illicit drugs for some time and had had amphetamine, methylamphetamine, cannabis and diazepam present in her body at the time of her death.

The judge recognised that the cocktail of drugs would have made her more susceptible to succumbing to the pressure on her neck and said that he was satisfied that Salcedo hadn't meant to produce the 'appalling consequences'.

Before passing sentence, he further commented, 'It is one of the least culpable cases of manslaughter in my experience on the bench.'

Dakohta Salcedo was subsequently sentenced to a minimum of two years with a maximum of four years.

Was justice served that day? It's difficult to say, so I'll leave that up to you the reader to decide.

9

'Cuppa Anyone?'

'To betray you must first belong.'
– Harold Philby

Flunitrazepam is a drug which has featured frequently in various drug facilitated sexual assaults (DFSAs) such that it became known as the 'date-rape drug'. Alarmed at the reputation the drug was getting, the drug company, Roche, changed the formulation to include a dye to warn of its presence in drinks and the Therapeutic Goods Administration (TGA) imposed further restrictions on the issue of drug, along with other potent benzodiazepine relatives such as Mogadon (nitrazepam). This was a case which involved a drink spiking using another brand of flunitrazepam (Hypnodorm) which unfortunately, at the time, did not contain a dye to warn of its presence in drinks. Here the motive was to incapacitate the victims and rob them, one whom was very wealthy.

★

It was a warm evening on 7 January 2002 when Ian Campbell invited Saylit Bulut (alias 'Eric') to his humble residence, a granny flat, for a casual visit.

They sat outside the granny flat and engaged in animated conversation on various topics. Eric later turned to Ian and asked if he'd like a cuppa.

'Yes, that would be nice,' replied Ian.

Eric then went into the flat and busied himself preparing their beverages, emerging minutes later with two steaming mugs of tea. Ian consumed the tea commenting to Eric that it was rather bitter.

'Oops, I forgot to put in sugar,' replied Eric.

Ian consumed the remaining tea and after some minutes started to become drowsy and lethargic.

'Come on mate, I'll help you into the flat.'

Eric then assisted Ian into his flat and laid him down on a couch. Ian by this time, was drifting in and out of semi-consciousness, before drifting off into a deep sleep.

In the meantime, Eric was busy assessing anything of value in Ian's flat.

Some 12 hours later, Ian awoke from his deep sleep drowsy, and also nauseous. It was a rude awakening. He discovered that his so-called 'friend' had stolen property to the value of $40,000, from his flat. He then contacted police and reported the crime.

Mr Campbell was taken to hospital where a sample of blood and urine were taken. The blood sample taken at St George Hospital at 3.30 pm the day after the incident was found to contain flunitrazepam 0.006 milligrams per litre. I found this level was quite significant given the long time interval, and suspected more than the therapeutic dosage had been given to the victim. (Also detected was the drug, nevirapine. This latter drug indicated that the victim was being medicated for HIV-1.)

But, Mr Bulut was still busy, and just over a year later he struck again.

At 8.20 am on the morning of 23 March 2003 Sayit Bulut visited a Thai transsexual (born a male, who had adopted the appearance of a female). With a similar modus operandi, he befriended the victim and offered 'Chris Nixon' (not her real name) a cup of coffee.

A short time later Chris slipped into an unconsciousness state and some seven-a-half hours later, awoke in a very drowsy state. In the meantime, a large amount of property in the form of jewellery, was stolen. Clearly, Mr

Bulut could not believe his luck; Chris was very wealthy and so he took advantage of the situation.

When Chris gained consciousness, it was discovered that the so-called casual 'friend' had stolen jewellery to the value of nearly two million dollars!

Police were promptly contacted and the crime reported. Ms Nixon was taken to hospital where a sample of her blood and urine was taken. The blood sample taken from Ms Nixon at 5.30 pm that day was found to contain flunitrazepam 0.006 milligrams per litre (mg/L). However, MDMA (ecstasy) was also detected in her urine. I found this level was quite significant given the long time interval, and suspected more than the therapeutic dosage had also been given to this victim. The presence of MDMA (3, 4–methylenedioxymethylamphetamine, ecstasy) in Chris's urine appeared to be puzzling at the time. Its presence may have accounted for the ease with which Bulut was able to befriend Ms Nixon – and administer the drug in her coffee. MDMA while being a stimulant drug, also tends to make the consumer more sociable and friendly, such that it has been called an entactogen or 'hug drug'. The street name ecstasy gives a hint as to its popularity in the social and/or 'rave' scene. However, no MDMA was detected in Chris's blood so it was difficult to determine whether this contributed to the victim's impairment!

The matter went before the district court in the presence of a jury. I was called to provide expert testimony in relation to the pharmacological effects of flunitrazepam found in the blood of both of the victims. I mentioned that flunitrazepam is a potent benzodiazepine-type drug that has central nervous system depressant effects, and that it produces a sedative effect, amnesia, muscle relaxation and a slowing of psychomotor responses with a rapid onset of action occurring some 20–30 minutes after ingesting the drug. However, the effects of the drug are long lasting.

I was further questioned, 'Doctor, in regard to the particular charges before the court, the allegation is administer a stupefying drug. Does this drug have the capacity to cause one to fall into a stupor?'

I replied, 'Absolutely. With only a milligram dose, the blood levels of flunitrazepam would peak at about 45 minutes after ingestion, and fall to one half after the peak after 20 to 30 hours.'

One victim clearly had more than this. The amount of flunitrazepam detected after 16 hours, was consistent with the ingestion of greater than a therapeutic dose of flunitrazepam.

Mr Bulut was found guilty and sentenced to seven years imprisonment.

Hopefully, by the time he is released he will have reflected on his former lifestyle and made appropriate amendments.

The Body in the Bay: Who Killed Katrina Ploy?

'Every unpunished murder takes away something
from the security of every man's life.'
– Daniel Webster

In the early hours of 18 December 2006, an abandoned dark-blue Hyundai sedan, registered to Ms Katrina Jessica Ploy, was found at the north face of The Gap near Watsons Bay, Sydney. Her belongings, including a white leather handbag, were found nearby, adjacent to the safety fence, directly in front of a sign warning of the dangers, along with a used cup of Starbucks coffee. But of the attractive and popular young lady, there was no sign. She'd last been seen alive by her parents at about 5 pm the day before, at their home in Seven Hills, in Sydney's north-west.

A week later, on Christmas Day, her body was found at Camp Cove, a short distance from Lady Bay Beach, Sydney. Her body had apparently drifted around the bay and subsequent wave action had washed it up onto the sandstone rocks, where it was sighted by a fisherman in a boat.

It's a mysterious death that up to the time of writing has remained unsolved. She was found clothed in a top and navy-blue coloured pants, the right leg of which had been rolled up as if she was planning to paddle in the surf. She'd obviously been in the seawater for some days, as there was slippage of her skin.

A post-mortem examination of Katrina's body was carried out on 28 December and revealed no fractures or serious injuries to any part of her body, nor any internal bleeding, which is inconsistent with a person falling, being pushed or being thrown from a boat or the cliff area of The Gap at Watsons Bay. She was believed to have drowned.

A blood sample taken from the body cavity at the autopsy was found to contain 3, 4-methylenedioxymethylamphetamine (MDMA) 0.36 milligrams per litre (mg/L) and alcohol 0.044 grams per decilitre (100 millilitres) of blood. The therapeutic range for MDMA in femoral blood is 0.10 to 0.35 mg/L, and within this range, the drug gives rise to an appealing combination of mild to moderate central nervous system stimulating effects, which in turn induces feelings of empathy, emotional closeness, euphoria, enhanced communication ability and changes in perception. The usual street dose is 75–150 milligrams, but with large doses exceeding this, amphetamine-like symptoms often predominate, including emotional lability, restlessness, increased heart rate, sweating, aggression, hyperpyrexia (elevated body temperature) and risk-taking behaviour.

However, Katrina's body was decomposing and cavity blood drug levels are not as reliable as femoral blood levels. Also, MDMA may exhibit post-mortem distribution, meaning the level detected could be higher due to tissue breakdown after death. Therefore, it was more likely her MDMA blood level at the time of death was within the therapeutic range, indicating recreational usage.

I reported that the MDMA concentration/s detected in Katrina Ploy's blood would appear to be consistent with a moderate ingestion of the drug. The presence of alcohol was most likely due to fermentation of glucose in her blood due to bacterial and/or fungal (yeasts) activity.

On 15 October 1996, when she was 19 years old, Katrina began her first job. It was as a clerk at Bellinger Instruments Pty Ltd, Rydalmere, Sydney. There, she met Nathan Shearman, fell in love and got married. They both later resigned from the company to start up a real estate business, but the marriage only lasted a short while due to ongoing domestic issues. After the divorce, Nathan made tracks for Townsville in Queensland and Katrina moved into a townhouse in Seven Hills. On 17 September 2003, she was brutally and violently assaulted by unknown persons inside her home, but nobody was arrested for the offence.

She then moved on to a residential unit in Parramatta, again living alone. On 28 January 2004, she recommenced employment at Bellinger Instruments Pty Ltd, while around the same time becoming involved with Joel Hollings from Century 21, a real estate agency in Seven Hills. They lived together for a period of time before the relationship ended in the middle of 2006. During that time, Katrina had further difficulties at her workplace, where she was apparently continually sexually harassed by the business manager and other colleagues. Seeking solace from her workplace troubles, she began dating Grant Millgate, an IT specialist. Millgate sympathised with her situation, saying, 'She was traumatised by work and trying hard to get out of there. You treat someone like a piece of meat for long enough and it damages them.'

Unknown to Katrina, she'd become involved with a man who had a criminal history, which included numerous traffic offences, as well as hindering the police. But as bad as that may have been, things were about to get worse.

Katrina used to go to a gym in Sydney, and while there, she was introduced to Adam O'Brien by Stephen Black (alias Stephen Pravdacich), one of Millgate's associates. O'Brien was a former Sergeant of Arms for the Bandidos Outlaw Motor Cycle Group and the owner of the Tattoo Nation tattoo shop in Wentworthville in western Sydney. He had an extensive criminal history with narcotics, in particular ecstasy.

He and Katrina developed a strong friendship, and his motor vehicle was often seen outside her residential unit complex prior to her death. He was also seen getting into his car shortly before she went missing. However, it's possible she'd been purchasing ecstasy from him as that drug turned up in her body. Katrina had also confided to her sister, Tania, that she wanted to get a tattoo, something Tania felt was amusing because it was so out of character for her to want to have one.

As for what Tania felt about Adam O'Brien, she said, 'If you'd asked me before, would Katrina have hung out with someone like that, I would have said "no", and it would have been a definite "no".'

But the connection between Katrina and Adam O'Brien was very close, as witnessed by the 50 calls she made to him in the month before she disappeared.

The inquest took place from 2 to 6 August 2010 at Glebe Coroner's Court in Sydney before Mr Paul McMahon, the deputy state coroner. The outpouring of grief by friends and family members during the proceedings laid testament to the fact that Katrina was a popular and much loved young woman.

Mr Warwick Hunt, the counsel assisting the coroner, opened proceedings by saying it was hoped that findings could be made into the time, manner and cause of Katrina's death.

'It must be said that there remain a number of possibilities available on the current evidence.'

I attended the inquest and was asked questions about the post-mortem tests that had shown Katrina had had the drug MDMA and alcohol in her system.

Mr Hunt asked if I was able to say what the likelihood of someone feeling suicidal after taking that type of drug was.

I replied, 'Folks take these drugs for the feel-good (euphoric) effect, so I think suicidal feelings would have been fairly unlikely.'

A number of other witnesses, including Sydney University physics professor Rod Cross also gave evidence at the inquest, suggesting that, 'It was possible that if Ms Ploy had taken a run-up to the cliff edge, she could have leapt in the water rather than onto the rocks.'

However, the minimal injuries sustained by the deceased didn't support that scenario.

According to Detective Sergeant Michael Kyneur, in a statement tendered to the court, in the two months prior to her death, Katrina had withdrawn more than $24,000 in cash from her bank account. Her boyfriend at the time, Grant Millgate, allegedly said that she'd made enquiries about having herself killed because she was unable do it herself. But he didn't know why she'd wanted to kill herself.

Those comments appeared to be somewhat doubtful, as Sergeant Kyneur said, 'Mr Millgate has shown a reluctance to be completely frank with information he's provided to police.'

Millgate also appeared reluctant to attend court, failing to appear on two occasions, thereby prompting the counsel assisting the coroner to request a warrant for his arrest, which was approved by Paul McMahon, the deputy state coroner, who said he was satisfied that Millgate had received a subpoena and that he'd provided no excuse for his failure to appear at court. Fortunately, for Millgate, he appeared the following Wednesday morning, so the arrest did not eventuate.

His evidence didn't appear to shed much light on the death of his former girlfriend, except when he said that Katrina had recently befriended a man, from then on known as Witness A, who not only had a reputation as a hit man, but who had also allegedly been supplying her with ecstasy.

On the final day of the inquest, Paul McMahon returned an open finding into Katrina's death, meaning the case isn't closed.

In summing up he said, 'I do not make a finding that Katrina's death resulted from actions taken from her intention of taking her own life. I am satisfied on the evidence that Katrina did not die as result of a fall from The Gap or endure any other 40-metre fall from any other location. There are numerous unexplained matters at this point. Some suspicion attaches to the death of Katrina.'

It was an unhappy result for her grieving family and friends, but there is someone out there who knows what happened to Katrina Ploy. If you have any information that may help put this case to rest, please call Crime Stoppers on 1800 333 000.

Down on the Farm: A Suicide

'While we are focusing on fear, worry or hate, it is not possible for us to be experiencing happiness, enthusiasm or love.'
– Bo Bennett

George Wiley and his wife Lucy had been married for 24 years. Like many other couples, they got along together quite nicely, with just the odd problem and occasional disagreement or argument. They lived in Wee Waa, a small country town in New South Wales, where Lucy taught at the local high school and George 'earned his crust' working the grape vines on their small farm, a short drive from where they lived. Every afternoon, George would go to the Royal Hotel and 'sink a few beers' and a number of Jack Daniels, more often than not becoming a little 'tired and emotional', something which annoyed Lucy and was the cause of most of their 'blues'.

One afternoon, late in March 2004, Lucy arrived home at her usual time of five o'clock and started to get an early dinner, as she was due back at the school for a Year 7 parent–teacher evening. George rolled in 30 minutes later and they spent several minutes enquiring about each other's day and generally having a pleasant chat. George cracked open a couple of tinnies and everything was going well. But then Lucy unwittingly dropped a bombshell.

'I was looking in the drawer where we keep the money to pay the farm workers and it doesn't all appear to be there. Do you know where it is?'

At first, George prevaricated, which made Lucy suspicious, although she didn't call him out, but a combination of her probing and his afternoon drinking quickly saw the situation escalate into a full blown war of words. Arguing about money was not new, but George's reaction to Lucy was more vigorous and unpleasant than normal.

'Well,' he growled, 'if that's what you think, piss off and go to your meeting. And if you reckon I spent the money, just watch me now.'

On that angry note, he left the house, got into his car and drove away.

Lucy continued preparing the dinner, expecting him to come back when he cooled down, but by the time she was ready to serve, he was still out.

When she returned from her meeting at around half past nine, the house was empty, so she assumed George had gone back to the Royal Hotel. Bedtime ticked round and he remained conspicuous by his absence. Not quite sure what to think, but a little worried, Lucy tried to rest, but spent a fitful night, waking from a light doze at 7.30 am the following morning.

George's side of the bed was empty, and a quick look around the house dispelled any hopeful notion she may have had about him being slumped on the sofa or in a chair. Lucy wondered if he'd possibly got so drunk he'd stayed at the Royal Hotel for the night, but then quickly dismissed the idea, thinking that it would be too out of the ordinary for him to do such a thing, and that if anything, he'd have stayed at the farmhouse. But whatever, she had to get to school, so with a heavy heart, she left the house and made the five-minute drive to work, where she signed in before putting in some time on her computer, catching up on administrative tasks, and going to the morning's assembly. After that, she had a meeting, and when she emerged at just gone ten o'clock, she was so worried about George that she approached the deputy principal and asked if she could take some time off to sort out a domestic problem.

The deputy principal was sympathetic and allowed her to go. First, she drove back home to check if George had turned up, but drew a blank, and then grabbed a pair of gumboots before driving to the farm, a couple of kilometres away. The boots were necessary, as recent rain had made the ground very muddy and it was difficult walking across the land without them. The gates to the farm were open when she arrived, so she drove in, only to be met by the excited barking of George's dogs, who, alerted by the sound of her motor, came running up to greet her. She saw George's car parked by the side of the farmhouse and felt an immediate wave of relief wash over her. But as she drew closer, she noticed the passenger door was open and that George was hanging out of the vehicle. Silly devil, she thought. He must still be asleep. How much did he drink to get in that state? But she wasn't angry, just pleased she'd found him.

She parked her own car, got out and went over. As she drew closer, she could see that not only was George positioned at a weird, rather unnatural angle, but that he was a purple-grey colour from his neck to his head. His trousers had also slipped down around his waist, exposing a band of white flesh and making his body appear longer than it really was. There was blood dripping from his nose, congealing on his moustache, and when she ventured to touch him, he was really cold.

'No, no, no!' she screamed, but there was no one to hear her pain and cry for help.

She took a few moments to compose herself before driving straight back to the school, where she told the deputy principal what she'd found. The police were called, and they, along with an ambulance, were quick to arrive at the farm.

After examining the scene and satisfying themselves that there had been no foul play, the police allowed George's body to be transported to the local mortuary. Then they turned to Lucy and started to question her as to the possible reasons why George might have taken his own life, drilling down on their financial situation.

Lucy told them that their finances were quite good and that they owned outright both the farm in Chifley Road, where George had been found, and their house in Warrior Street. She also told them where she worked and how much she earned. Expanding further, she admitted that the 2003–04 grape harvest had been less than hoped for due to the poor weather, and that the money they would be receiving from that year's harvest would be a lot lower than for the previous year. When pressed about debts, Lucy replied that although they often argued about expenditure, there were no debt problems. The police were satisfied with what she told them, especially as they'd be able to verify everything she'd said, and ruled out money as a reason for her husband taking his own life. But the question remained: Why did he do it?

It was hoped that the post-mortem might be able to shed some light on the matter.

A blood sample taken showed the presence of 5.05 milligrams per litre of arsenic, which is well above the average level of 3.3 milligrams per litre (range: 0.6–9.3 mg/L) normally found where there has been an intentional or accidental overdose.

George had clearly ingested sufficient amounts of the toxin to do its destructive work, resulting in his death. An additional blood sample showed a blood concentration of venlafaxine 0.3 milligrams and alcohol 0.108 grams per decilitre (100 millilitres of blood). Venlafaxine (Effexor) is an antidepressant drug which works by inhibiting the reuptake of certain neurotransmitters, including serotonin and adrenaline, in the brain – and, hopefully, maintaining the brain chemistry so that those levels can be maintained. Unfortunately, alcohol at elevated levels can interfere with those desired outcomes.

Further post-mortem observations showed there was face bruising to the upper and lower eyelids; conjunctiva multiple haemorrhaging to both eyes; some blood clotted around the mouth and nose; multiple bruising to the neck (front), shoulders and both arms; cyanosis of both ears, the fingernails and the toenails; multiple small haemorrhages in the area of the larynx and on the vocal cord, and the back of tongue was very blue and congested, although there was no evidence of obstruction.

Whether George meant to take his own life or not will never be known for sure. He was known to suffer from depression, hence the venlafaxine, and together with the alcohol he'd been ingesting all afternoon, his judgment and thought processes might well have been impaired, leading him to take the arsenic. However, that is purely conjecture, and the only thing that can be said for certain is that his wife truly cared for him and for a row to have provoked his subsequent actions is just too sad to contemplate. There really was no worthwhile motive or reason for George's demise.

Stricken by Strychnine

'All that counts in life is intention.'
– Andrea Bocelli

Strychnine is an alkaloid derived from the disc-shaped seeds of the evergreen strychnine tree (*Strychnos nux-vomica*), which is indigenous to the tropical and subtropical climatic regions and grows in abundance in South-East Asia, India and Australia. It's a potent central nervous system stimulant and convulsant, which acts through the selective blockade of post-synaptic neural inhibition. Essentially, that produces the tetanus–like symptoms that are observed with this poison. It's been widely used as bait in the control of vermin, especially for the extermination of rodents and predatory animals such as foxes. In adult human beings, death, which is truly unpleasant, may occur after the ingestion of 60–100 milligrams due to either asphyxiation caused by the paralysis of the respiratory muscles or exhaustion from the resultant convulsions.

Strychnine is rapidly absorbed from the gastrointestinal tract, with half of the dose being distributed to the tissues in about five minutes. There is an onset of symptoms within an hour, during which time, all the muscles of the body contract simultaneously, leading to the characteristic convulsion. This can become so extreme that the body arches and only the heels and the crown of the head of the person suffering the awful effects remain in contact with the ground. The facial muscles also undergo a tetanic spasm that gives rise to the *risus sardonicus* expression of the features; a face so contorted that most people find it difficult to forget.

★

The morning of 16 December 2009 was warm and sunny. At 'Wotcmajig' farm, Ian Johnstone and his son, 10-year-old James, started to wash up after their breakfast. Ian's estranged wife, Sue, had left for work sometime earlier at 7.30 am. Their marriage had been undergoing difficulties, with him suffering from depression and her having a thyroid complaint to add to their woes, and they were officially separated. She'd moved out of the family home some time previously, but a few days earlier, she'd decided to move back in temporarily to finalise property and custody issues. While there, she helped out with the everyday household chores and duties, one of which was the administration of Combantrin, a worming medication, to their two children. It was a necessary precaution to take given the family's close proximity to the farm animals, and was common practice in rural areas. On that particular occasion, she'd given the children their doses the previous evening, when she'd also taken hers, leaving Ian to have his the following morning. As he swallowed the regulation three spoonfuls of the medication, he pulled a face and said, 'Yuck! This is awful.'

Not long after, while still at the sink, he felt a great pain stabbing in his chest. Clasping his hands to his body, he wheezed, 'Son, I need help. Call an ambulance.'

His son tried to use the phone, but it wasn't working, so the valiant lad ran 4 kilometres to his grandmother's home, where he called 000 for help. While he was gone, his eight-year-old sister remained with Johnstone, who continued to bang and thump his chest in pain.

An ambulance arrived at about 10.35 am, by which time Johnstone had collapsed, foaming at the mouth. The ambulance officers started resuscitation efforts and were able to take him to Inverell Hospital. He was unconscious when they arrived and still wearing a blue rubber washing-up glove on his left hand. The big problem was that a spasm had caused his jaw to lock and they were unable to get a clear airway. Despite frantic medical attention, Johnstone was pronounced dead shortly after arrival at the hospital. He was only 38 years old.

His body was transported to the Newcastle Department of Forensic Medicine on the morning of 17 December 2009 for a post-mortem by Dr Allan Cala at 9.30 am the following day. The post-mortem examination failed to establish a cause for his chest pain, as his heart was observed to be normal. No significant coronary artery narrowing was identified, nor was there any evidence of aortic dissection or pulmonary thrombo-emboli. Essentially, his heart showed no apparent diseases.

However, a toxicological analysis of a blood sample taken from Johnstone at the post-mortem showed the presence of strychnine and a small quantity of the antidepressant, citalopram. I requested that those substances be quantified. There was also a small amount of grey fluid in his stomach, but that, unfortunately, was not submitted for toxicological analysis because at the time of the autopsy, given the verbal evidence of events, his death was suspected to have been from natural cardiac or respiratory causes. It would have been a very useful sample to test, and would have been helpful in subsequent enquiries.

A further toxicology report revealed that a blood sample taken at the post-mortem was found to have present citalopram less than 0.1 milligrams per litre and strychnine 7.0 milligrams per litre.

Citalopram is available under the trade name Celexa, which may have been prescribed to treat Johnstone's anxiety and depression. However, Loxalate was found among his medications, and that contains escitalopram (a pharmacologically active 'cousin' of citalopram), which is also used to treat depression. Interestingly, there was no Combantrin. I concluded that the concentration of strychnine in Mr Johnstone's blood was well into the lethal range to result in his death.

So, how did the strychnine get into Ian Johnstone's system? The possibility of the poison being mixed with the worming preparation

Combantrin was raised because pyrantel pamoate (the active ingredient in Combantrin) and strychnine are both quite bitter in taste, so could a lethal dose of strychnine have been mixed into the Combantrin suspension?

Strychnine is generally found in a powder form. It comes in several colours, ranging from off-white to pale pink. Initial thinking was that it might not be possible to mix the powder into the suspension, as it might turn into a paste, so a mixing experiment was carried out to test if it was feasible. A 55 ml bottle of Combantrin oral suspension was purchased from the local pharmacy and three doses of 15 ml (about three teaspoons) were measured out into three glass beakers. The beakers then received 120 mg, 260 mg and 347 mg (– half a teaspoon) respectively of the pale pink strychnine powder (>95% pure as the sulphate) before being briefly stirred with a glass rod. All three doses mixed readily into the Combantrin, with minimal, if any, residue being observed.

I concluded that it was possible to mix in very toxic to lethal doses of the strychnine powder into a recommended dose of Combantrin oral suspension. No noticeable colour change was observed after mixing, and minimal residue was observed after disposal.

The inquest into Ian Johnstone's death took place in Inverell on 8 September 2011. The coroner was Michael Holmes. The court was told that on the day Ian Johnstone died, Laurence Burdekin (also known as 'Scrubber'), Johnstone's best friend, met Sue Johnstone at the hospital after being informed of his death. Many of Ian Johnstone's friends and family said they believed that the two had been romantically involved long before his death. Sue Johnstone denied that, saying she and Burdekin only became close after her husband's death. Yet, within weeks they were an 'item', and a year later they got engaged and moved into the family home where Ian Johnstone had died.

Detective Anthony Esham told the court that police suspected that either Sue Johnstone, Laurence Burdekin or both may have been involved in his death. However, they also had an alternative explanation, suggesting that Johnstone may have taken his own life, as he'd attempted to gas himself in 2007.

After interviewing Sue Johnstone and the two children, detectives formed the theory that the poison had most likely been in a bottle of Combantrin, something the mixing experiment had shown to be possible, but the problem was that no bottle of Combantrin had been found in the house, a matter which had become central to the case.

As a consequence, the coroner concluded, 'Ian Johnstone died as a result of strychnine poisoning, but I am unable to determine the manner in which the poison was administered.'

Detective Sergeant Anthony Esham said the file would remain open and hoped new information would help to solve the case.

Readers are encouraged to call Crime Stoppers on 1800 333 000 with any information that may assist investigators in this case.

The Case of Mercury in the Ice Cream

'That was the best ice cream (soda) I ever tasted.'
– Lou Costello

Although mercury does have poisonous properties, particularly when in finely divided form (for example, 'blue mass' preparations, which are so called due to the colour produced) and when heated to produce a vapour, metallic mercury intoxications are very rare. At ordinary temperatures and pressures, mercury is a liquid metal, and because of that, its high density (13.53 grams per millilitre) and its electrical conductivity, it's a very versatile metal. Generally safe, it's used in a vast array of applications, including barometers, sphygmomanometers (early devices used to determine blood pressure), wall thermostats for heating and cooling, batteries and electric switches. However, it has been known for some accidents to occur.

★

It was mid-June in 1996 when Peta Smith purchased a 2-litre tub of ice cream for her family as a treat. She took it out of the shop freezer, paid for it at the checkout with her other purchases and went home, where she placed the tub in the freezer compartment of the family refrigerator. The following day, her husband, Jack, took the ice cream out of the freezer and helped himself, his daughter and young son each to a portion of the ice cream, together with some canned black cherries and custard. He then replaced the lid of the tub and put it back into the freezer.

Unfortunately, the ice cream was contaminated with metallic mercury, something he and his family were to become only too aware of later that evening. The first one affected was his son, who complained of stomach pains and started to cry, but not thinking anything was amiss and fancying some more ice cream, Jack once again took the ice cream out of the freezer and scooped some into a bowl. It was only after he'd eaten a couple of spoonfuls that he noticed a silver bead at the bottom of his dish. After attempting to remove what he thought was a solid object, it broke into a number of smaller beads, and it was at that moment he realised it was metallic mercury. He alerted his wife and took the ice-cream container out of the freezer. They poked about in it with a spoon and found it was riddled with silver globules.

Peta clutched her hand to her chest in horror. 'Oh, my God, we've been poisoned with mercury!'

Wasting no time, the family piled into their car and drove to the casualty department of the local hospital, where Jack and the two children were seen by a doctor, who ordered X-rays, blood tests and urine samples to be taken. He also took X-rays of the ice cream tub and its contents, which Jack had had the presence of mind to take with them.

The federal police were also notified, and suspecting it to be a case of deliberate poisoning, they took further photographs of the ice-cream tub.

Jack and his two children were given a laxative and released from hospital that same evening, at the same time being advised to return if they experienced any health problems.

Unfortunately, the attention they received turned out to be just 'band aid' treatment, as the doctor didn't consider metallic mercury to be poisonous. While he was correct up to a point, he should have taken into account the fact that the more finely divided most metals are, the more active they become, which was what had happened to the mercury.

This particular phenomenon is essentially due to the larger surface area provided by the metal, it becomes more reactive when it's in a divided form. A familiar example is iron. Iron nails become red hot when exposed to a flame, but a more divided form, such as steel wool burns.

Later that night, Jack experienced severe headaches, stomach cramps and very bad diarrhoea, while his daughter also suffered with the latter two symptoms. But for Jack, that was just the beginning, as he not only became excessively irritable, but also started to experience difficulty recalling if he'd completed tasks and forgot appointments (short-term memory loss). In some cases, he couldn't remember how to perform familiar work processes. There was clearly a serious problem.

And matters got worse. He began to encounter difficulty picking up small objects and using familiar work tools, such as a screwdriver. That was accompanied by a feeling of exhaustion after limited effort. He also became confused easily and felt that nothing was real. As a result, his personality started to change, including a seething anger towards himself for the problems he felt he'd brought upon the family.

He feared he was going to die and leave his wife on her own to care for the children, and whenever he heard or read anything sad, he'd become over emotional and even start crying. He said he had a constant feeling of being uptight and sad at the same time, and that although he felt lonely, he didn't want to be with people.

His symptoms appeared to be consistent with mercury poisoning, mercury being a neurotoxin (a poison that affects the nervous system). Its effects were first noted in the nineteenth century amongst hat makers or hatters, who were exposed to mercury in the felting process (mercury was incorporated into the material to preserve it), leading to frequent outbreaks of mercury poisoning, which in turn gave rise to the term 'as mad as a hatter'.

Symptoms of mercury poisoning include personality changes, such as mood swings, and becoming irritable, frightened, excited or depressed for no apparent reason. Loss of memory and the ability to concentrate may also occur. Other health effects include a form of gingivitis and kidney damage.

It was bad enough Jack and his two children being exposed to mercury in the ice cream at all, but it was made worse because the mercury was in a finely divided form, thereby not only making it more active and improving the metal's absorption into the body, but also exacerbating its toxic effects.

On page 1053, under the heading 'Mercury and Mercurials', *Martindale: The Extra Pharmacopoeia* (26th edition), 1972, by William Martindale states: 'When applied locally in a finely divided state, mercury is absorbed through the skin and was formerly employed by inunction in the treatment of syphilis and chronic skin diseases.'

Jack went on to see nine more doctors or other health professionals over the course of the next seven years, which might on the face of it seem somewhat excessive, especially if one considers that even President Lincoln didn't seem to need so much treatment after experiencing toxic effects from the blue pills he'd been prescribed (they were pills that contained mercury in a finely divided state). But, in Jack's case, the amount of mercury he'd ingested was unknown, even though there was a consensus of opinion between the professionals that he visited that his symptoms were consistent with mercury poisoning.

He began a series of chelation treatments, starting with mercury reducing drugs, using penicilliamine, and monitoring mercury levels in urine. Chelation (derived from the Greek khele or claw) is a technique for removing heavy metals from the body. This is achieved by using chelating drugs, which essentially grasp the heavy metal atom in a chemical claw and thus expedite its removal from the body. The technique proved to be successful and gave Jack some relief from his devastating health symptoms, but not before the detrimental effects on his career, family life and overall health had set in.

In time, he approached a law firm in an effort to get some compensation through the due process of law, after which he hoped to be able to get on with his life.

The Supreme Court of the Australian Capital Territory is the superior court for the ACT and has unlimited jurisdiction within the territory in civil matters. It hears the most serious criminal matters, and it was there that justice was sought for Jack against the manufacturers of the ice cream.

Prior to the Supreme Court listing, I was consulted by Jack's barristers on several occasions regarding the effects of mercury poisoning, and I examined the various certificates, documents and X-rays to do with the offending ice cream, including a report from the University of Sydney where the ice cream had been further analysed to establish the level of mercury present.

At the time, it seemed to me that the poisoning had probably occurred as a result of a most unfortunate accident, such as a broken thermostat spilling its mercurial contents into a tub of ice cream while it was cooling. However, the major flaw in that line of thinking was why hadn't one of the workers reported the problem of a broken thermostat or similar mercury containing device to their supervisor or manager? But, there is always the possibility of human error.

In the Supreme Court, I was cross-examined at length on the properties of mercury and its effects on the human body. Given the rarity of elemental mercury poisoning, the devastating health consequences of exposure to the metal are quite often not recognised, and this case proved to be no exception, so it took some convincing evidence and the presentation of a number of published cases to show the court that some of the mercury was in a finely divided form in the product.

The judge weighed the evidence presented by me and a number of other experts, deliberating over the matter for some time, and he eventually found in favour of Jack, with the manufacturer of the ice cream being held liable for what had happened. At first, that appeared to be a good result, but unfortunately, the judge didn't accept that the effect of the mercury poisoning could have gone on for as long as it had and that it had only lasted a few days, a conclusion not supported by the peer-reviewed literature and Jack's medical records. Subsequently, Jack was only awarded the sum of $10,000 plus costs.

He had his day in court, but whether or not he received justice, I'll leave that for you the reader to decide.

Brave Heart:
Police Officer Down

'Show me a hero and I'll write you a tragedy.'
– F. Scott Fitzgerald

Located in the New England region of New South Wales, Tamworth is a delightful country town that straddles the Peel River. It's situated almost midway between Brisbane and Sydney. In the 2011 census, the urban centre of Tamworth was recorded as having a population of 36,131.

The town is known as the First City of Lights, being the first place in Australia to have electric lights, in 1888. It's also famous as the country music capital of Australia, hosting the Tamworth Country Music Festival, the second largest country music festival in the world, every January. And if that isn't enough, the town is recognised as the national equine capital of Australia due to the number of equine events held there, a number unparalleled anywhere in the Southern Hemisphere. Tamworth is undoubtedly a top place to live in New South Wales.

★

It was just another routine day on Friday 2 March 2012, when at 6 am,

40-year-old Senior Constable David James Rixon, a father of six, began duty at Tamworth's Oxley Local Command as a highway patrol officer.

He climbed into a fully marked white New South Wales Police Ford Falcon sedan, with the call sign Oxley 203, and headed off to the Gunnedah Highway, west of Tamworth. Between the time he left the station and 7.30 am, he was quite busy, attending to a non-serious motor vehicle accident and a number of vehicle traffic stops for random breath tests.

At about 7.50 am, Michael Allan Jacobs pulled into a Caltex service station in his 1996 white Holden Statesman to purchase petrol and a packet of cigarettes. With the transaction completed, he left the station a few minutes later and drove out onto the Gunnedah Highway, heading towards Tamworth town centre. Senior Constable Rixon noticed the vehicle and a quick check with the onboard computer revealed that the driver was disqualified from holding a New South Wales driver's licence, along with other details of his motor vehicle. At the time, Rixon was travelling in the opposite direction, so he had to make an abrupt U-turn, at which time he activated the in-car video recording system. This useful device records both visual events and sounds, along with conversations, making it a great evidence gatherer for the prosecution in the case of any subsequent court action. As a back-up, portable microphones are also carried by highway patrol officers, which have also proven to be excellent sources of evidence. This case proved to be no exception.

Senior Constable Rixon followed the unlicensed driver to a block of units in Lorraine Street, Tamworth, which was Jacobs' home address. At about 8 am, Rixon alighted from his vehicle and turned on his portable microphone.

As he approached the vehicle Jacobs was driving, in true Australian fashion, Rixon said, 'G'day mate, how you going?'

'Not bad,' Jacobs replied.

'Just going to breath test you, buddy.'

As Rixon passed over the breathalyser, Jacobs reached for a loaded .38 calibre Smith & Wesson and fired, hitting him in the chest, the bullet passing through his heart and lung. Chillingly, Jacobs then said,

'Die! I'm sorry, sorry, sir,' which was picked up on the Rixon's portable microphone. In the meantime, Rixon, although he was mortally wounded, reached for his Glock, and in an act of extraordinary courage, fired off four shots, incredibly, hitting Jacobs in the leg, abdomen and shoulder. Then, amazingly, he still managed to reach out and partially handcuff Jacobs before collapsing unconscious onto the ground.

On hearing the shots, a long-term Tamworth resident somewhat bravely jumped out of her bed, grabbed a dressing gown and dashed across to where the gunfire exchange had taken place. She saw Rixon lying face down on the ground, and another man on his side, facing the flats. She went straight up to Rixon and rolled him over to see if he was still breathing. He was, so she asked him to keep breathing and placed him on his side. Then she turned her attention to the other man and noticed a black pistol close to where he lay. She asked his name.

He moaned and said, 'Michael Jacobs and my shoulder hurts.'

'Why did you do it?' she asked. 'Why did you shoot the police officer?'

But Jacobs just groaned in pain from his injuries.

Meanwhile, police and ambulance personnel had been alerted, and they arrived on the scene shortly after. CPR was performed on Rixon, but despite the ambulance crew's best efforts, he was declared dead by the time he arrived at Tamworth Hospital.

Jacobs, however, survived his injuries and was conscious. While the police were completing his handcuffing, he said, 'I'm sorry, I'm sorry … I've been shot, I've been shot!'

He was treated by paramedics and taken to Tamworth Hospital, where, after emergency surgery, he survived.

Strike Force Fairfull was subsequently instigated to investigate the incident.

A blood sample taken from Michael Jacobs while in Tamworth Hospital was found to contain methylamphetamine 0.18 milligrams per litre (mg/L), amphetamine less than 0.02 mg/L, morphine 0.10 mg/L, midazolam 0.008 mg/L and methadone 0.23 mg/L. No alcohol was detected.

Given his injuries, morphine and midazolam were expected to be found, as they'd been administered by hospital staff at 9.05 am on the morning of the incident.

The methadone was within the therapeutic range and indicated that he was on a drug rehabilitation program. However, the main player was the stimulant, methylamphetamine. The therapeutic range for it (or methamphetamine or just meth) in blood is 0.01 to 0.05 milligrams per litre. Within that range, the drug has an appealing combination of mild to moderate central nervous system stimulating effects. However, levels well above that range (depending upon usage and tolerance) can result in increased wakefulness, increased physical activity, decreased appetite, increased respiration and hyperthermia. But worse, the drug can impair a user's faculties by altering perceptions and judgement and increase aggressive or risk-taking behaviour. And if the levels are high enough, the drug may also produce hallucinations.

Jacobs' blood level of methylamphetamine was just over three times the top end of the therapeutic range. It had clearly affected his behaviour.

Because a police officer had been killed, the matter became a very high-profile case.

Many witnesses appeared during the subsequent month-long trial at the Supreme Court, Darlinghurst to give evidence, including me. From the outset, Jacobs pleaded not guilty to the crime. His defence barrister, Mr Tim Hoyle, SC, suggested that someone else may have been responsible for the shooting, claiming that Terrance 'Terry' Price (a known drug dealer) had been the killer.

Barrister Hoyle suggested to Terry Price that he'd arranged to meet Jacobs for a heroin deal and had been about to hand over the drugs, when Senior Constable Rixon had appeared on the scene. 'You said to [Jacobs], "What's the fucking cop doing here?" And with that, you pulled out a gun and you shot the police officer.' Hoyle then suggested that rather than Jacobs shooting Senior Constable Rixon, he'd tried to wrestle the pistol from Price, only the police officer had shot him three times, at which point Price had fled from the scene.

Price replied, 'That's the first time I've heard that.'

Price denied any involvement in the shooting and said he'd been in bed at the time with his girlfriend, Monica Sampson.

However, Price did possess an unsavoury record, having previously served almost eight years in jail for a 2003 manslaughter when he'd stabbed a drug dealer to death in a dispute over a $150 drug payment and a mobile phone.

Price also denied any suggestion that he'd 'acted spontaneously' and shot the police officer because he'd feared being found with drugs.

Further evidence was presented that showed gunpowder residues had been found on Jacobs' hand and a DNA profile matching his had been detected on the .38 calibre pistol. The same tests on Price proved negative.

The defence were clearly clutching at straws.

Further evidence was presented by the crown prosecutor, Pat Barrett, from a conversation that had been secretly recorded as Jacobs had been recovering under guard in hospital. In it, he told his girlfriend, Sharon Strudwick, several things, including, 'I wish I hadn't have had the gun, wish I hadn't have got the shits that morning. I've been like it all my bloody life, get the shits over nothing.'

Taking methylamphetamine (meth) would not have helped the situation.

Sharon Strudwick was cross-examined and said she'd found a black box containing bullets in the garage of the apartment she shared with Jacobs, in the days after the shooting. Unfortunately, she had told her son, James Strudwick, to hide them up a toilet pipe moments before the police had come to search her premises. (That incident was to later lead to further charges.)

I was subsequently questioned at length about the methylamphetamine detected in Jacob's blood and its effects, and said that it would 'have contributed to increased aggressive and risk-taking behaviour.' However, I concluded with, 'But he would have been well aware of his actions.'

It appeared fairly clear-cut to me from the outset that the offender (Jacobs) had been under the influence of methylamphetamine, although given the levels detected, he could still have functioned and still carried out the foul deed.

Eventually, when all the evidence had been presented, Jacobs was found guilty.

Unfortunately for him, laws introduced in 2011, a year before the offence, required judges to impose a life sentence on any offender found guilty of murdering an on-duty police officer. In sentencing Jacobs to life in prison, Justice Richard Button said, 'It is almost impossible to believe that, in order to avoid a short period of being denied bail or, at worst, a sentence of a matter of months for driving whilst disqualified, the offender saw fit to fire a handgun at a police officer. The murder of a police officer in such circumstances is a direct assault upon our system of parliamentary democracy and the rule of law.'

Importantly, Justice Button found that Jacobs' offence met all the criteria that were set out in the mandatory life sentence legislation, including the intention of killing the officer with a previously loaded weapon.

He went on to further say, 'That the intention may have been held only fleetingly and uttered irrationally, but nevertheless I consider that it has been established to the criminal standard. The result is that the mandatory life sentence is to be imposed.'

With that said, and in a landmark decision, Michael Alan Jacobs, 49 years of age, became the first person to be sentenced to life in prison under the new laws requiring a mandatory life sentence for anyone who murders an on-duty police officer in New South Wales.

Having made the six-hour journey from Tamworth, almost a quarter of the Oxley Local Area Command were present, and they formed a guard of honour for Senior Constable Rixon's widow, Fiona Rixon, and her six children as they left the court.

A very emotional Mrs Rixon said, 'I'm very proud of my children. We've been through this hurricane, tornado and roller-coaster ride, whatever you want to call it, for the last 18 months. Now hopefully, life will be a bit more quiet.'

However, more was to follow.

Sharon Strudwick was later charged with acting with intent to pervert the course of justice after pleading guilty to interfering with the police murder investigation. She said she'd only been trying to protect herself and her son when she'd told him to stash the box of bullets down a toilet S-bend, and was only sentenced to 20 months jail, with a 10 month non-parole period. Given public sentiment at the time, she was quite fortunate that the sentence was not more severe.

Senior Constable David Rixon's death touched everyone, particularly those who serve within the police force, who never know when a dangerous incident may occur, and his fellow officers wanted to honour their fallen comrade in a special way.

On the morning of 7 March 2012, roads were closed and traffic disrupted as Tamworth stopped to mourn the tragic loss of one of their own. A full police funeral took place, including marching escorts, hundreds of police colleagues and a roadside guard of honour, which was formed outside St Paul's Anglican Church in Church Street, West Tamworth. The procession to the church included police cars (one marked with the number plate 'Rixon'), motorbikes, a police band and police on foot.

I was quite touched, as were many others. It was a huge turnout.

Police aircraft (Polair helicopters) also joined in a salute from the air, and many politicians, including NSW Premier Mr Barry O'Farrell, attended, along with representatives from the NSW ambulance services and NSW fire brigades. The latter were helpful in assisting the network of road closures and maintaining order during the consequent traffic disruptions.

The NSW police commissioner, Mr Andrew Scipione, read the valedictory alongside a eulogy for the Rixon family, and Senior Constable Rixon was awarded posthumous medals for courage (BM) and valour (VA) for 'conspicuous merit and exceptional bravery whilst under fire.'

The police commissioner commented, 'It's never easy to say goodbye to someone who meant so much to so many.'

Superintendent Clint Pheeney of the Oxley Local Area Command, where Senior Constable Rixon worked, said, 'I think it will be a time to mourn and grieve with the family of David and all our colleagues over his tragic loss. It will also be a time to remember the contribution he's made to the community and the NSW Police Force.'

It was a moving ceremony, and due to the number of people attending the service, it was also streamed onto big screens outside the church. After the service, family and close friends of Senior Constable Rixon attended their own private burial service, away from the considerable media glare.

Ms Jemma Galea, the stepdaughter of Fiona and David Rixon, was in the final stage of studying to enter the police force when her stepfather was gunned down. Andrew Scipione kindly offered her the option to postpone her studies while she dealt with loss of her father, but the young woman, although grateful, was resolute, saying, 'I want to make my father proud.'

A year later, she delivered, and the then Probationary Constable Jemma Galea joined in a charity walk in honour of her father on the anniversary of his death.

She wore a bright pink cap bearing the police force insignia, as it had been something of a personal joke between her and her stepfather. She explained, 'David said to me when I bought it, "When are you ever going to wear that hat?" So, now I wear it, to remember him.'

Finally, a plaque honouring Senior Constable Rixon was unveiled by Andrew Scipione during a ceremony marking the anniversary of the tragedy, at the Tamworth Community Centre.

A fitting tribute.

The Black Widow: A 'Morphine Mistress'

Bill, 'Have a nice rest.'
– Kerry Forrest

As a forensic investigator, from time to time, I've been involved in cases of extraordinary human treachery that have sometimes left me quite speechless. This case was no exception.

★

Kerry Forrest (née McGregor) was born on 20 September 1959 to a lower middle-class family. At 15 years of age, she set out on her life of crime with several stealing charges, appearing before Minda Children's Court, where she was committed to six months' institutional care for each offence. She then 'graduated' with a false pretences charge and appeared before Albion Street Children's Court in Sydney, where she was fingerprinted and spent further time in institutional care. From then on, there was a continuous string of charges, ranging from stealing from dwellings to various fraudulent acts, with appearances before courts such as Parramatta Petty Sessions, and later, Windsor Court of Petty Sessions. In addition, she committed a number of traffic offences, including displaying a misleading registration label.

She subsequently changed her surname to Jewel, and it stayed that way until she met Wayne John Forrest, who she married after getting out of jail, when she took on the name Kerry Forrest. They had two daughters, Kisha and Kara, but normal domestic life was never on the cards, and a number of scams, including several fictitious assaults for compensation, eventually led to divorce and Wayne Forrest remarrying his first wife, Gail.

But Kerry was only just getting started. The stage was now set for the big one – a financial venture that was to dupe William 'Bill' Adamson, a recently widowed war veteran. He was 84 and his 90-year-old wife, Beryl, had passed away in September 2009 from Alzheimer's disease.

His first contact with Kerry had been in 2002, on the internet, where he ran a business called Australian Rain Saver. Kerry expressed interest in purchasing one of the products on offer, and over the years, she told Bill that she was 'going through a bit of a hard time with her husband'. They struck up a friendship and he would ring and ask if she was alright. At that stage, the relationship was purely platonic with no other involvement.

Prior to Beryl's death, Bill had employed two health care workers to look after her; one was a qualified nurse and the other was a carer. After she died, they were no longer needed, but he still wanted a companion to cook his meals, wash his clothes, do some ironing and carry out some housework, so he advertised the position through Seek, an employment agency. At the same time, Kerry wanted to leave her allegedly abusive husband and was searching for work. She saw Bill's advertisement for a live-in carer, and noting that appropriate qualifications weren't considered necessary, as the duties were considered purely domestic with no medical issues involved, she jumped at the opportunity, and Bill was happy to welcome her aboard the 'good ship Adamson'. (Given the number of cases I have been involved with over the years where vulnerable old folk needed help, this problem needs to be addressed.)

It appeared to be a mutually agreeable arrangement and Kerry promptly moved into the Kareela property, where she was provided with a self-contained granny flat. They settled into a routine, with Kerry apparently also receiving some government benefits as a carer to Bill.

Before long, a joint bank account was set up, a strong indication that the relationship was clearly becoming more intimate than that of employer and employee, and then Bill put his house up for sale. It was never clear why, except maybe for him to have sufficient money to buy a waterfront property, because his business was based in the Kareela house and it had been home for him and Beryl for many years. Also, it was not far from Oyster Bay, various parklands and many other local facilities. All in all, it was a very nice location in south Sydney.

Not surprisingly, given the location and the Sydney property boom at the time, the property sold quickly. So quickly, in fact, that Bill and Kerry had to find alternative accommodation in a hurry and storage for the furniture and various household goods. Some were even stored in an adjoining neighbour's property.

Apparently, the plan – or at least what Bill, a former realtor and property developer, thought it was – was to build a house on a plot of land that Kerry owned in Bundanoon, a town located south-west of Sydney. Bill's house sold for $690,000, leaving a profit of $319,000 after fees and commissions. That was duly deposited into their joint account, which was subsequently transferred to Kerry's account on 12 April 2010. In the meantime, they had a pressing need for temporary accommodation.

They packed their immediate possessions, along with Bill's medications, into the boot of a 1993 Lexus sedan and headed off to Campbelltown, an outer suburb of Sydney, to stay at the Maclin Lodge Motel, which Kerry had previously booked because it was close to her daughter, Kara, who lived in nearby Camden. The room was well-appointed, containing two queen-sized beds and a large flat-screen television, but curiously, Kerry had only booked it for a week and paid cash up front at a $110 a night plus a further $50 for the key, a total of $820.

At 6.35 pm on the evening of Monday 12 April 2010, Bill and Kerry moved into room 58. The first couple of days were uneventful, with Kerry going to Woolworths to get some hot chicken and other food items. Then on the evening of 14 April, Bill decided to go to bed early, as he was very tired, and began to snore quite heavily. While he slept, Kerry placed a 'Do Not Disturb' sign on the door, later giving as a reason the fact that a woman had 'barged in' while she and Bill had still been asleep in their beds the previous day. On the morning of 15 April 2010 she left Bill in the room, but not before placing a note, written on Maclin Lodge Motel paper, behind a plastic jug.

> *Bill,*
> *Gone to MOVIES & SHOPS & to do all the things*
> *you wanted me to do.*
> *Will be home very late.*
> *I will try to be very quiet.*
> *Have a nice rest.*
> *Love Kerry*

When she returned in the early hours of Friday 16 April, Bill was still lying in the same position on the bed. It was plain that he was dead and had been for some time. Kerry then contacted Dr Tan Mao, the family doctor, hoping that she would come to the motel room, examine Bill, pronounce him deceased and issue a death certificate, thus avoiding a police investigation. But unfortunately for Kerry, Dr Mac had other commitments and said she couldn't go to the motel, whereupon Kerry, quite inexplicably, drove to the doctor to collect Bill's medical records. She then returned to the motel and later telephoned 000 at about 10.50 pm. The police arrived soon after, and the stench of death was only too apparent.

A crime scene was set up and various items and medications were photographed before being removed for later forensic examination. Bill's body, after being photographed in situ, was taken to the Glebe mortuary by government contractor Russell Illingworth of Statewide Mortuary Transfers. Meanwhile, Kerry went to Campbelltown police station and was interviewed.

Although she wasn't under arrest, she was interviewed for some hours and asked various questions as to what had led to Bill's death. She was very keen to distance herself from it, saying that she'd got back Friday afternoon at about 4 pm and found him 'stone cold' and believed he'd died in his sleep from 'extreme exhaustion.' However, she'd waited until nearly 11 pm before calling the police. That irregularity was further explored during the interview, but she was insistent that everything had been normal and that 'he just fell asleep with the telly on' while he was in bed and that she'd previously gone out to purchase food.

Her stories were starting to become very inconsistent. Further questions were asked.

'Do you know how he died?'

'In his sleep.'

'Do you know what may have caused him to die?'

'I have no idea.'

'Were you involved in his death in any way?'

'No.'

The interview terminated at 2.20 am and Kerry was allowed to head back to the motel, which she checked out of the following day, preferring to stay with her daughter, Kara.

She now had a sizable bank account of over $300,000, and was no doubt looked forward to spending it, but she had a serious gambling habit, and within three months, she'd gambled the lot away on poker machines. Gambling, unlike drinking or smoking, has no limits. Too much alcohol or too much nicotine kills. End of story. But gambling goes on and on. While there's money, there's a bet.

Effectively, there was nothing left of Bill's estate for his stepson, John. It was a sad outcome for a worthy next-of-kin. However, investigators were still busy on the case and were awaiting the post-mortem and toxicological reports from the death.

Bill Adamson's body arrived at the Glebe Department of Forensic Medicine during the evening of 17 April 2010 and the post-mortem was carried out at 9 am on 20 April by Dr Isabella Brouwer. It was apparent that the body of the elderly man was 'in an early state of decomposition with extensive autolytic changes (breakdown of tissues) in the organs'. Other than that, it presented as that of a well-nourished elderly male with no serious health issues.

However, the toxicological analysis of a post-mortem preserved blood sample was found to contain a morphine (free) level of 3.8 milligrams per litre and an alcohol level of 0.010 grams per 100 millilitres of blood. In addition, promethazine (Phenergan) was detected. The morphine was the main subject of interest, as being well into the lethal range, it had clearly resulted in his death.

Bill was not known to drink alcohol and none had been brought to the motel, so the detection of a small amount of the substance in his blood was no doubt due to bacterial and/or yeast fermentation of the glucose in his blood, as his body was showing signs of decomposition. Also, the detection of promethazine was not unexpected, as some Phenergan medication had been found in his satchel of medication at the motel. It had been used to treat his skin allergies.

Promethazine also has potent anti-emetic and anti-nausea properties, which can prevent the nausea/emesis that can occur with high doses of morphine.

Phenergan would have assisted the absorption of the morphine and prevented vomiting occurring, thus ejecting the poisonous dosage administered to Bill's body. No morphine medication was found in his personal possessions, but an almost empty foil pack of MS Contin (morphine sulphate) was found in Kerry's possession, although she had been prescribed them for her own pain. Senior Constable Anthony Holmes was keen to link the morphine tablets to her, and so I suggested comparing an isotopic profile of the morphine in the tablets to the morphine found in Bill's blood. However, that complicated procedure proved unnecessary, as the foil pack only had Kerry's fingerprints on it.

In any case, I concluded in my final report that the elevated blood concentration of morphine, along with the presence of promethazine, was more than sufficient to depress Mr William Adamson's respiratory system to the extent that life was unsustainable.

With that evidence, it became a clear case of murder and Strike Force Human was formed to investigate. It began by monitoring Kerry Forrest's activities over the course of several months. In the meantime, she'd been busy moving around the state, eventually taking up a property under an assumed name. Shortly, after she'd settled into her new accommodation, she was arrested and charged with murder. It was the evening of Valentine's Day, 14 February 2011.

Life is full of ironies.

She appeared before Bega Local Court the following Tuesday 22 February, where she was formally charged and refused bail. She also had a number of driving offences outstanding, including driving while disqualified, driving an unregistered and uninsured vehicle and displaying a misleading registration label. But those paled in comparison to the murder charge, which was adjourned to Campbelltown Local Court on 6 April. The driving offences, being less serious, were put-over for a two-day committal hearing over 22 and 23 August 2012.

Given the very high level of free morphine (3.8 milligrams per litre) detected in Bill Anderson's blood, I thought it prudent to have the total amount of morphine determined. That meant re-analysing the blood sample for bound morphine (the amount attached to the blood proteins) as well as the free morphine, or essentially, the total amount of morphine. The reason for doing that was that it would not only provide a way to establish how much of the drug had been inadvertently consumed by Bill Adamson prior to his death, but also present a means to determine approximately how long it had taken him to die from the effects of the drug by looking at the ratio of the free drug in relation to the total amount as a percentage.

The result came back at a whopping 11 milligrams per litre of morphine, which proved to be very useful evidence to be presented in court. With that information, I was able to give an estimate of the amount of drug consumed and an approximate length of time it had been taken before Bill Adamson's respiratory system had shut down from effects of the drug, thereby taking his life. In this case, it was 34.5%, and the higher the ratio percentage, the shorter time of death.

I was questioned at length about the pharmacological properties of morphine and the various ways that the drug can be taken into the human body. Then, predictably, I was asked about the amount of time it would have taken the deceased to die. I told the court that according to my calculations, 'death would have been in excess of three hours. If it was closer to 50 per cent, well, that indicates a much shorter period of time of death. So as you get the larger percentage the faster the person has passed away.'

Further questions were raised, including the number of 100-milligram MS Contin tablets Bill Adamson would have needed to consume to reach the morphine blood levels observed. I had earlier provided an estimate based on the free morphine figure. That proved to be very conservative, and I said to the court, 'I was relying mainly on the 3.8 milligrams of free morphine. Now, that was just an estimate and I said even this estimate may be conservative. Well, once I got the other analytical result of 11 milligrams per litre, and that's total morphine, it certainly indicated that my estimate was very conservative. So, based on that, I would indicate that it would have been greater than 10 tablets that had been consumed.'

Prior to my evidence, Dr Olaf Drummer from the Victorian Institute of Forensic Medicine had also given his expert opinion via an audio-visual link to the court. It appeared we agreed on most of the issues, except for the number of MS Contin tablets consumed. His estimate of 'more than two tablets' was even more conservative than mine. Even though Bill Adamson had weighed only 64.5 kilograms at the time of his death, it had to be much more than two 100-milligram tablets! Nevertheless, after further police evidence was presented, the court found that sufficient evidence had been supplied to take the matter to the Supreme Court.

On 17 March 2014, the matter was subsequently heard before a judge-only trial, with Justice Peter Hidden presiding. Kerry Forrest, now 54, was brought into court in a wheelchair. She was wearing dark sunglasses and her head was bowed. It was a pathetic sight, and whether the scenario was for sympathy, or a genuine medical condition, only time was to tell. She waved briefly to her daughter, Kara, as she took her seat in the witness box.

Asked about the proceeds of the sale of the Kareela house, Kara told the court her mother had wanted to use the money to build a house in partnership with the elderly man, adding, 'We visited some display homes in Kellyville.' She said not long after that, her mother had turned up at her Camden home, saying that Bill Adamson had died. 'She said that Bill had passed away and I asked if she had reported it. She said, no, she hadn't. She then went to the bathroom and splashed water on her face.'

She then related how Kerry Forrest had explained to her that she'd been out all day and that when she'd returned to the Maclin Motel where they were staying, she'd found him dead. It was then that she'd asked Kara and her boyfriend to call the police and ambulance, and to drop her around the corner of the motel.

Questioned about her mother's gambling problem, Ms Forrest said it was so bad that after Bill Adamson's death, she'd caught her playing two poker machines at once and had to confiscate her debit cards.

Further evidence was provided by Detective Senior Constable Cate Fuller, who told the court that when she arrived at the motel room, she found Bill Adamson deceased and a case that had a large amount of medications in it. She also said that when she asked to search Kerry Forrest's bag, she became 'upset and defensive', and on searching the bag, she found Bill Adamson's wallet, along with his cash, health and credit cards.

The court also heard that Kerry Forrest had moved the proceeds of the sale of the Kareela property to her own bank accounts only days after Bill Adamson's death.

I was the last witness, and appeared on a fairly bleak, rainy day, which pretty much set the mood of the proceedings dealing with the death of an elderly war veteran. The questions put to me were very similar to those at the earlier Campbelltown Local Court hearing and so the answers were the same. However, the judge was curious as to how Kerry Forrest had managed to get Bill Adamson to ingest so much morphine that it resulted in his death. I don't like to speculate and prefer to deal with hard scientific facts, but I could understand where he was coming from, as it was a lot of one drug, and a bitter one at that, to consume.

MS Contin is a sustained release dosage of morphine sulphate that is formulated to give patients relief from pain over an extended period of time. To get a rapid release and the high levels of morphine detected in Bill Adamson's blood, the tablets would have had to have been crushed up. But morphine, and indeed the opiates in general, are very bitter, so the taste needs to be disguised. I suggested that the drug powder could have been mixed into a beverage that was already bitter, such as coffee. But who knows, other than Kerry Forrest, whether the toxic dose of the powder was also mixed in other food she offered to Bill Adamson in his final hours.

In any case, the judge was satisfied that Kerry Forrest was guilty of the murder of William Adamson, having crushed up the tablets, possibly 10 or more, before feeding them to him, possibly in his coffee.

In his summing up, he said, 'Ms Forrest misappropriated Mr Adamson's money and killed him to prevent that misappropriation being exposed.'

It was a sad end for a veteran who'd fought for Australia, only to be murdered decades later by a woman who posed as his carer.

On 27 November 2014 Justice Peter Hidden, after much deliberation, sentenced Kerry Forrest to a maximum of 25 years in jail, with a 19 year non-parole period. As she'd already spent nearly three years behind bars since her arrest in February 2011, she would be eligible for parole on 13 February 2030.

However, while in Long Bay prison, she'd been diagnosed with cervical cancer, along with several other serious medical conditions, which had left her in a wheelchair – hence the court appearance.

Justice Hidden conceded that the minimum term was 'well beyond her life expectancy' of six to 18 months, given her medical conditions and that the cancer was considered incurable. However, he said it was not in his power to consider an early release. Only the state government and state parole authority could direct an early release in exceptional circumstances.

So Kerry Forrest was effectively given a life sentence for murdering an elderly man to support her gambling habit. Whether her cancer is truly incurable and her other medical problems treatable, only time will tell.

Death of a Brave Firie

'A hero is no braver than an ordinary man,
But he is braver five minutes longer.'
– *Ralph Waldo Emerson*

With very dry weather, hot summers and bushlands of gum trees rich in very combustible eucalyptus oil in their leaves, Australia is a bushfire-prone country. It's only ever a lightning strike, a misused flame or worse still, an arson attack away from a fiery disaster. And it's in such situations that our brave firefighters, more affectionately known as firies, swing into action. They are one of a number of professions (including those to which this book is dedicated) that literally put their lives on the line to protect people and property. They are heroes in the true sense of the word.

★

Philip Viles, a self-employed upholsterer and devoted husband and father of three children, was a part-time firie, joining the fire brigade as an on-call firefighter 14 months before the incident in this story occurred.

Part-time firefighters never know when they're going to be called to duty. Although, the onset of warm, dry conditions heightens the general fire risk and provides some indication a call won't be far away. However, not all call-outs relate to bushfires. Some are for suburban fires, which result from various sources such as flaming cooking oil, faulty electrical wiring and children playing with matches.

And so it was on 26 July 2004 at 1 am, that a call was received informing the fire station that a home in Denman Street, Doyalson, New South Wales was ablaze. Flames were tearing through the building, weakening the structure of the two-storey house and threatening a young family. The Budgewoi and Doyalson fire teams sprang into action and fought their usual valiant fight, rescuing most of the family before debris started to fall, the ceiling started to buckle and the air became so full of thick choking smoke, it was impossible to see.

But just when the firefighters thought the worst was over, the rescued 33-year-old mother screamed, 'My little two-year-old son is still in there.'

He was trapped in the upper storey of the house.

Downstairs, Philip Viles donned his breathing apparatus and tried to make his way up to the second floor to rescue the child. Falling masonry was everywhere, and the intense smoke and heat hindered his progress. But he never gave up and tried several times to reach the boy. However, each time he was rebuffed by the searing heat and ever thickening smoke, which was growing more poisonous by the minute as various vinyl fabrics and other combustibles were consumed by the flames, adding cyanide and carbon monoxide to the already deadly fumy mixture.

Viles returned to the outside of the building, where he collapsed through sheer exhaustion. He was immediately treated by paramedics and transported to Wyong Hospital. But it was to no avail. He was dead on arrival.

It took the firefighters a further hour to bring the blaze under control, and sadly, the two-year-old child, Brent Londrigan, perished in the blaze. It was a terrible and tragic outcome after so much effort had been put in.

Phillip Viles' body was taken to the Newcastle Department of Forensic Medicine on the morning of 27 July for a post-mortem, which was carried out by Dr Kevin Patrick Lee at 11.50 am the following day.

The post-mortem showed that Phillip Viles' 'trachea and major bronchi had somewhat inflamed mucosal surfaces. Their lumina contained a moderate amount of mucus with a little inhaled food material. The lungs were of unremarkable configuration. Their pleural surfaces were unremarkable apart from moderate carbon blackening.'

Those findings indicated that Viles may have inadvertently inhaled partially digested food material (in the form of vomitus) and that he had been exposed to smoke, which may have come from smoking and/or his firefighting duties. However, more importantly, his heart was not in good shape.

'The main trunks and major branches showed severe atheroma. The left common artery showed up to 80% occlusion in its middle and distal parts. This included some calcification but was mainly fibroatheroma with a little part-organised pale surface thrombus. The left anterior descending branch showed 70–80% occlusion over long segments in the form of fibroatheroma and calcific disease. The left circumflex branch showed 50–70% occlusion by fibroatheroma and calcifying disease. The right circumflex and right posterior descending branches showed 40 and 30% occlusion respectively over short segments with fibroatheroma.'

The pathological findings were severe coronary artery disease and terminal inhalation of vomitus.

The subsequent toxicology report of the blood samples taken from Viles at the post-mortem stated that his blood contained carbon monoxide 5% saturation, cyanide ion 0.1 milligrams per litre, delta-9-tetrahydrocannabinol (delta-9-THC) 0.014 milligrams per litre and delta-9-THC acid 0.032 milligrams per litre.

The level of carbon monoxide was relatively insignificant and was most likely derived from smoking cigarettes and some smoke inhalation while Viles had been performing his firefighting duties. That conclusion was supported by the presence of cyanide ion in his blood, which was most likely derived from a number of sources, including organic cyanides from burning plastics such as acrylamide (vinyl) products that had been metabolised in the body to the cyanide ion.

However, the level of delta-9-tetrahydrocannabinol (delta-9-THC) was of interest. A level of 0.010 milligrams per litre or greater provides presumptive evidence of recent consumption of cannabis (or marijuana), but it isn't possible to determine exactly when it was consumed. Even so, such a level would be expected to produce some impairment in a person's abilities to carry out various tasks.

In my conclusion, I opined that, Mr Phillip Viles passed away through an existing health condition, which may have been brought about by strenuous activity.

Philip Viles was given a hero's send-off on Friday 30 July in the Central Coast town of Noraville. Hundreds of people lined the streets and gathered inside St Mary's Catholic Church to pay their final respects to one of their own, a brave firefighter.

In a moving eulogy, Fire Commissioner Mullins said, 'Phillip Viles was a true hero. A hero to his family, a hero to his community and a hero to the men and women of the NSW fire brigades and our fellow emergency services. It is one of the saddest ironies, that while Phil was known for his big heart, it was tragically his heart that gave out on Monday night. I can't claim to understand why, in this double tragedy, we lost one of our most promising firefighters, and the life of a two-year-old child. It doesn't make sense. I do know that Phil and other firefighters did everything they could to rescue little Brent Londrigan. I also know that when Phil collapsed after the frantic rescue effort, the paramedics and firefighters did everything they could to save their colleague. Most importantly I know that Phil died as he lived – putting other people first.'

After the service, Viles' coffin was conveyed to a nearby cemetery by a NSW fire brigade hearse, complete with a police motorcycle escort and the accompaniment of bagpipes and the Budgewoi band.

At the graveside, his sons placed various items associated with the seaside he'd loved, while members of the Budgewoi Brigade each placed a yellow rose on his casket.

Commissioner Mullins said, 'We say goodbye to a husband, a father, a son, a brother, a firefighter, and a good mate. Most importantly, we say goodbye to a true hero.'

Phillip Viles was posthumously awarded a Commendation for

Meritorious Service medal for his firefighting efforts, while two of his colleagues, Station Officer Denis Raynor and Senior Fire Officer Philip Brown, received medals for conspicuous bravery. Viles' award has only been given to 27 firefighters in the fire brigade's 120-year history. Superintendent Ian Krimmer said that fighting the fire had taken its toll on Viles, 'He continued to make gallant efforts until he collapsed and died.'

The incident didn't pass unnoticed in the New South Wales Parliament, where the topic, 'Death of Retained Firefighter Phillip Viles' was raised by the Honourable Jan Burnswoods, who said, 'My question is addressed to the Minister for Emergency Services. What is the Government doing to protect the families of New South Wales firefighters in the event of workplace deaths or injuries?'

The Honourable Tony Kelly replied, 'In recent weeks, we have again been reminded, in the most tragic circumstances, of the courage and dedication of our State firefighters. Not many professions require individuals to risk their lives to save others who are in danger. But our firefighters face that risk every day, and they do so with great bravery and a staunch spirit.

'Those who make up the ranks of fire services deserve our highest praise and collective gratitude. In particular, today I want to pay tribute on behalf of every member of the Parliament and the community of New South Wales to retained firefighter Phillip Viles.

'Honourable members would be aware that on 26th July, firefighter Viles lost his life in a valiant attempt to rescue two-year-old Brent Londrigan from his burning home at Doyalson on the Central Coast. I understand that Brent was the son of a worker in the corrective services department. I am sure that all honourable members will join with me today in extending our condolences to both the Viles and the Londrigan families at this difficult time. The loss of both Mr Viles and young Brent was a blow to their families and friends, as well as the small community in which they lived. The fire brigade's colleagues of Mr Viles are also, understandably, devastated by the loss of one of their own. The firefighting community is close knit and the death of a member, especially in such tragic circumstances, is felt very deeply.

'Phillip Viles had been a firefighter for only 14 months, but he was recognised as one of the fittest and most committed members of his brigade. His captain, Bruce Simpson, said that whenever there was a call-out, "Phil attended them and was always the first there. That sort of dedication is pretty rare." His family and friends said that Phil would have shied away from being called a hero. That may be so, but there can be few other descriptions of a man who repeatedly braved flames and choking smoke to try to save a small child's life. Those who spoke at his funeral painted a picture of a good bloke, a joker, a keen surfer, a man who loved his boys and a hero. I can only echo the view of Fire Commissioner Mullins, "If we measure a man's life by what he leaves behind, I'd say he's a great man, a legend."

'Mr Viles leaves behind his wife, Tracey, and his three sons Joshua, Luke and Matt; three young boys who will now grow up without their dad at their side. Although nothing can bring him back to them, at the very least they will be supported financially under the fire brigades' death and disability arrangements.

'The New South Wales Fire Brigades' Firefighting Staff Death and Disability Award 2003, which came into effect in March last year, guarantees that should firefighters be killed or injured, they and their loved ones will be protected financially. The New South Wales fire brigades' firefighters now have the most comprehensive death and disability coverage in Australia. As a result of this award, firefighter Viles' family will be entitled to a significant lump sum workers compensation benefit. They also will receive a fortnightly pension. I am aware that the community and a number of corporations have rallied to support the Viles and the Londrigan families, as has his local brigade.

'This has been a distressing incident for all involved. Our thoughts remain with all of them. I cannot pay high enough tribute to our firefighters for the job they do and to Mr Viles who, in doing his job, paid the ultimate price.'

Unfortunately, the consumption of a joint of cannabis may have given Philip 'five minutes longer' to brave the awful fiery situation, but it was a double-edged sword, as it also compromised his abilities to deal with the various exertions involved in firefighting, and given his health situation, it may have contributed to his sad demise.

Albeit a heroic one.

Psychosis and a Case of Patricide

'Schizophrenia cannot be understood
without understanding despair.'
– R. D. Laing

This was a most unusual case. Most of the cases I've dealt with over the years have involved offences that have occurred while under the influence of various drugs, whether legal (licit) – for example, alcohol – or illegal (illicit) – for example, methylamphetamine. Here, the perpetrator was suffering from a lengthy mental illness, which was controlled by several medications. However, because the medications appeared to have either been taken in insufficient amounts, or worse, not to have been taken at all, psychosis took over with deadly effects, and so the tragedy occurred.

★

Shamin Fernando was born on 16 July 1967, in Sri Lanka, and migrated to Australia with her family four years later. She had two other sisters, Dayanthi and Michelle, and enjoyed a normal childhood. When she reached her early twenties, she unfortunately began to suffer from schizophrenia and a major depressive disorder. Not too surprisingly, those medical conditions impacted upon her working life, wellbeing and personal relationships. Nevertheless, with medical care and appropriate medications, clozapine (Clozaril) and venlafaxine (Efexor – XR), she was able to maintain a normal life, even completing a degree in communications at the University of Technology, Sydney, and landing a job managing a community radio station associated with Macquarie University.

However, she started to become reluctant to take the medication, in particular, clozapine, saying to her mother, 'If I accept that I have got this illness, I'll never be able to trust my own judgment again.'

But due to her mental health, she had a strained relationship with her father, Vincent 'Lalin' Fernando, even with the medication. To further complicate matters, she began to self-medicate and became a heavy user of cannabis. Excessive cannabis use is known to exacerbate an underlying psychotic condition. She became somewhat delusional, thinking there was a global conspiracy against her, organised initially by a former university lecturer and later by her father. Worse still, she believed she was under surveillance and that her personal information was being broadcast while the details were being withheld from her.

As for her father, he was very loving towards all his children and was eager to seek a reunion with Shamin. But mental illness doesn't reason in the usual way, and she perceived her father as a serious threat.

In preparation for dealing with the 'conspiracy', she joined the Sydney Pistol Club at La Perouse, a suburb in south-eastern Sydney, after filling out an application form and providing two character references. No mention was made of her mental illness, and she checked the section referring to that condition as 'no'. She now had access to a firearm and plenty of ammunition.

At 9 am on Sunday 22 August 2010, Shamin went to the Sydney Pistol Club in order to carry out some target practice on the range. She signed out a club-owned .22 calibre Ruger semi-automatic pistol and bought two boxes of ammunition, each containing a hundred rounds, from the club's duty officer, George Petas, a firearms dealer. She then joined in the 'match of the day' and fired off 70 rounds of ammunition during the session. After the session finished, she hid the weapon in her handbag, along with remainder of the ammunition, before leaving the firing range.

At 1.45 pm the same day, Shamin returned to her one-bedroom unit at 12/2 Victoria Road, Glebe and loaded six bullets into the magazine of the Ruger pistol, which she placed under a quilt on the bed. Then she called her father on both his mobile phone and home landline, leaving messages for him to call her. 'Dad, I need help to load some software now, please ring me back.'

At 2.19 pm, she eventually contacted him and repeated her request. Thinking it could be the beginning of a reconciliation, her father was eager to assist. 'Yes, of course, what time?'

'Oh, about three will be fine.'

Meanwhile, the pistol club's gun-keeper, Patrick Slavik, had noticed that the gun signed out to her hadn't been signed back in according to the club's regulations, but he thought it was a clerical error and that the gun had been returned, only realising it hadn't been when he went to put the guns from the day's activities into a locker. Now worried, he phoned the club captain, who called the secretary to check Shamin's details in the gun register. The secretary then tried unsuccessfully to call her at 2.42 pm.

Shamin's father arrived promptly on the hour at the Glebe unit and was ushered into the lounge room, where the computer was sitting on a desk. He pulled up a chair and commenced work, loading disks into the system. While her father was busy, Shamin went to her bedroom and pulled the loaded Ruger out from under the quilt. She then opened the bedroom door and moved into the lounge, where she aimed the pistol at the back of her father's head and fired off five rounds. The first shot misfired, but the other four hit him. He stood up and cried out in pain before staggering towards the kitchen, where he collapsed. Not sure whether he was dead or not, Shamin went back to the bedroom and loaded more rounds into the pistol, returning to the lounge and firing a further three rounds into the twitching body. The execution was complete.

Shamin then sat down and contemplated the situation for a while, wondering if the neighbours had heard and if they would call round. But nothing happened, so at 3.14 pm, she called 000 and asked for the police, saying she'd just shot her father in the back of his head and he was now dead. Just two minutes earlier, the pistol club captain had called police to tell them that she'd stolen a gun from the club.

The police arrived shortly after and the first police officer on the scene, after establishing they were at the right address and that he was talking to Shamin, shouted through the door, 'Just step out of the flat with your hands up and walk out backwards.'

Realising the situation she was now in, Shamin yelled, 'I'm walking out backwards now and my hands are up in the air.'

As she emerged, a further instruction was barked, 'Get on your knees!'

Shamin duly dropped to the floor and was asked where the gun was.

'On the sideboard.'

But the police, not knowing the situation fully, weren't taking any risks, so they handcuffed her and she was taken down to police headquarters.

In the meantime, an ambulance arrived with paramedics, and after assessing that Vincent Fernando was dead, took his body to the Glebe mortuary, not far from where his delusional daughter lived.

As with most police investigations, and particularly serious offences, a strike force was initiated. This one was called Strike Force Simmie. At about 6.30 pm that day, Shamin was interviewed via ERISP (Electronically Recorded Interview of a Suspected Person) at the police station in Newtown.

An ERISP is a police procedure whereby a person being interviewed is recorded both on audio and video. The general legal advice in such a situation is that they only give their name, address and date of birth, but should not answer any further questions until a criminal lawyer is contacted. A document titled Caution and Summary of Part 9 of the *Law Enforcements Act 2002* is read to the interviewee prior to the session.

On legal advice, Shamin initially decided not to say anything. However, after being asked if she was happy to be interviewed about the shooting, she answered in the affirmative. The usual procedural questions were then asked before the interview moved on to the events of the afternoon.

'What was the purpose of him [Vincent Fernando] coming around? When you made the phone call, what were you thinking?'

'I wanted to shoot him.'

'So why did you ask him to come round and load software on your computer?'

'If I asked him to come round so I could shoot him, I don't think he'd come.'

Then, chillingly, she chuckled at the thought.

Further questioning dealt with how she managed to remove the gun from the pistol club undetected, how and when the gun was loaded and where the gun had been stored prior to the killing.

Asked why she'd joined the pistol club, she replied without hesitation, that she'd wanted to get a firearm to 'shoot the old man'.

Finally, the questioning came down to the motive for the killing.

'Why did you want to shoot your father?'

It was here, under further questioning, that it became evident that Shamin was quite delusional. She said that she was trapped in a reality-style TV show and that her father was the main producer. It involved being monitored by hidden cameras and the show was broadcast on the internet and television. It also required her to pretend that it wasn't happening and that her thoughts were actually psychotic delusions, meaning she had to take medications, see doctors and not to discuss the show or the production. Essentially, she felt trapped in this Truman-like show that was supposedly orchestrated by her father, and she thought the only way to get out of it was by killing him. 'Yeah, shooting the old man was the only way out.'

Someone once said, 'There is no reality, only perception', and in this case, a loving father was unfortunately perceived as a manipulating television producer trapping his daughter into a pseudo reality-style TV show.

Further from reality, it would be hard to get.

Given the seriousness of the offence, the matter went before the NSW Supreme Court and Justice Peter Hall on 15 December 2011.

The court was told that members of the Sydney Pistol Club rang police at 3.12 pm on 22 August 2010 to report the missing Ruger gun, just two minutes before Shamin Fernando rang police to confess to having shot her father. The court also heard that Shamin lured her father to her Glebe unit on the pretext of getting him to load software onto her computer. However, the main issue raised was how a probationary gun club member had been able to take a weapon away from the pistol club so easily.

A further issue raised was that of mental illness, as Shamin had crossed 'no' by the question on the club form that asked whether she had any mental illness preventing her from using a firearm safely, and there had been no checking of the information she'd provided.

My evidence was rather brief. I said, 'I am of the opinion that at the time of the incident, given the symptoms described of Ms Shamin Fernando, they would appear to be consistent with her untreated medical condition said to be paranoid schizophrenia. However, it appears a blood sample was not taken at the time, so it is not possible [for me] to determine whether she was adequately treated for her medical conditions or not.'

But the previous evidence given by other witnesses indicated that Shamin's mental illness had not been adequately treated.

After considering the evidence, Justice Hall found that because of her mental illness, 44-year-old Shamin Fernando was not guilty of murdering her 70-year-old father. However, she was remanded in custody under section 38 of the Mental Health Act until such time that psychiatrists determine she is fit to be released. Until then, she will receive treatment at the Forensic Hospital at Long Bay.

Shamin's mother, Carmen, while grieving over the incident, said that her daughter was not a criminal. 'She's a victim, just as we are. This happened because she was inadequately treated and because of the access she was given to a firearm despite being seriously mentally ill.'

Following the shooting, the NSW Commissioner of Police, Mr Andrew Scipione, tried to suspend all shooting activities at the Sydney Pistol Club, but was prevented from doing so by an Administrative Decisions Tribunal, which said the club had tightened its regulations and that closure of the facility would adversely affect its 150 members and put the club's survival at risk.

However, the instructors at the pistol club failed in their duty of care.

Subsequently, George Petas and Patrick Slavik were prosecuted. Petas was found guilty of selling ammunition to an unlicensed shooter, although no conviction was recorded, while Slavik was found guilty of failing to supervise Shamin Fernando and failing to keep a firearm in a safe place. He was fined for both offences.

Since the tragedy, Shamin's sister, Michelle, a criminal lawyer, has been on a campaign to tighten a loophole in the gun laws. She believes that a weakening of the NSW firearms laws in 2008 was partly responsible for her father's death. She cannot understand how her mentally ill sister managed to walk out of the Sydney Pistol Club with a semi-automatic handgun along with an estimated 130 rounds of ammunition in her handbag.

After the Port Arthur massacre, where 35 people were murdered, the then prime minister, John Howard, brought in laws to ensure that anyone possessing and shooting a gun had to be licensed. Unfortunately, the Shooters Party brought in an amendment (6B) to the NSW Firearms Act in 2008, which was supported by the Labor government under Bob Carr at the time, which allowed people aged 12 years and older to enter a gun club and shoot without a licence. Furthermore, shooters were no longer required to wait 28 days to permit a police background check for a criminal record, domestic violence or mental illness.

A spokesperson from the police minister's office said, 'Labor, under Bob Carr, made several changes to gun laws that were a betrayal of the Howard government's National Firearms Agreement.'

Asked whether the minister was comfortable with 12-year-olds shooting at gun clubs, he replied, 'We are comfortable with the resources of the NSW police force deployed through the NSW Firearms Registry to ensure that shooting is carried out safely and under supervision.'

In true politician-speak, he effectively ducked the question.

Despite the shooting and killing of Vincent Fernando and a change in government, the 2008 change to the Firearms Act unfortunately still stands.

Not a good result.

The Pill Popper and the Copper: A Car Boot 'Pharmacy'

'It was for my own use, I suffer from hayfever.'
– accused drug dealer

I regularly received cases that involved clandestine laboratories making methylamphetamine from ephedrine and the more readily obtainable pseudoephedrine. The police called them 'pseudo runners'. However 'pseudo' means false, so it's probably not a good choice of words.

But run they did, all along the eastern coast of New South Wales, with those responsible stopping off at one pharmacy to buy a few packets of drugs containing pseudoephedrine before moving on to the next. Unfortunately, this network has now spread throughout the state.

Pseudoephedrine is readily converted into the more valuable (and much more potent) methylamphetamine (more commonly known as meth, methamphetamine) using a number of chemical methods, one of which is known as the iodine and hypophosphorous reaction, although there are a number of other procedures also used for this chemical conversion.

People who have this knowledge and know how to extract this drug precursor from various pharmaceutical preparations such as Demazin are known as 'cooks' and are in much demand by so-called bikie gangs, who distribute the final product. I would prefer to call them chemical 'crooks', but more of that later.

★

On the afternoon of 2 November 2005, Allan Michael Harvey was driving along the Newell Highway in a southerly direction from Gilgandra, a distance of just over 67 kilometres from Dubbo, New South Wales, with two other male passengers. Harvey had a minor criminal history in Queensland and had been unemployed for the past two years, having apparently found another way to earn a living. Shortly before 1 pm, the Dubbo police received information about the activities of the occupants of that very motor vehicle, which told them they were not regular tourists. As a result, they conducted a patrol along the highway, and waited.

Shortly, after 1.10 pm, the suspected vehicle was sighted travelling about 20 kilometres north of Dubbo. The police pounced, stopping the vehicle, and spoke to the driver, Allan Harvey. He was told that he and his fellow passengers were suspected of having purchased quantities of pseudoephedrine tablets for illicit purposes. Harvey was asked if he would permit a search of his vehicle, which he did, signing a police notebook to that effect.

The police officers searched the boot and found three carry bags containing personal items. Two of the bags belonged to the male passengers. Of interest, was a large sports-type carry bag, which Allan Harvey indicated was his. On opening the bag, a large number of resealable plastic bags containing small light blue tablets were found, along with other plastic bags containing larger darker blue tablets. The plastic bags were marked in handwriting '6 hour' and '12 hour'. A further search of the sports bag revealed further resealable plastic bags, several of which contained small amounts of white powder, together with a glass case, which had another plastic bag containing green vegetable matter (euphemistically known as gym or cannabis).

The police had stumbled upon a veritable 'pharmacy' in the boot of the vehicle. But there was more to come!

A further search of the vehicle revealed a cloth zip-up bag under the driver's seat. The bag had a further nine blister sheets containing 36-hour Demazin tablets and two sheets holding 18 12-hour Demazin tablets.

In all, the police found 240 small blue tablets (Demazin 6-hour tablets), 54 large blue tablets (Demazin 12-hour tablets), nine blister sheets of 6-hour Demazin tablets, totalling 270 tablets, two sheets of 12-hour Demazin tablets, totalling 36 tablets, and three small plastic bags of white powder (amphetamine), plus a small amount of cannabis.

Investigating police conducted a number of enquiries and it appeared that Harvey and his two mates had been very busy over the previous 48 hours. The information received showed the trio had visited a number of pharmacies, purchasing Demazin tablets in the townships of Moree, Narrabri, Coonabarabran, Gunnedah and Gilgandra on their way to Dubbo. Harvey was arrested, cautioned and taken to the Dubbo police station, together with the cache of tablets and other drugs (now seized as police exhibits) that had been found in the motor vehicle. (It's not known what happened to his two accomplices.) In addition to the drugs, police also discovered a large sum of money (in excess of $3000) tied in separate bundles. One can only speculate about the probable use of the money, but it was highly unlikely to have been earmarked for the purchase of a motor vehicle, as suggested in the subsequent police interview.

Following various legal and police formalities, Harvey was taken to the ERISP (Electronically Recorded Interview of a Suspected Person) room, and after being cautioned about his rights, he was interviewed. On being questioned, he freely admitted to possessing cannabis and the bags of loose tablets found in his bag. But, quite incredibly, he said the tablets were to treat his hayfever – 600 tablets!

Pseudoephedrine is used as a nasal and bronchial decongestant, and when combined with an antihistamine drug such as dexchlorpheniramine, as in the Demazin formulation, it provides effective temporary relief for sinus and hayfever conditions, as well as for cold and flu symptoms. The usual dosage of pseudoephedrine is 60 milligrams, twice or thrice daily (that is, 120–180 milligrams per day). Therefore, 600 tablets containing a total of 41.4 grams (or 41,400 milligrams) of pseudoephedrine sulphate would represent between 230 and 345 days' supply, which is almost a year, assuming one to one-a-half tablets are taken daily. Larger doses of pseudoephedrine may give rise to undesirable side-effects such as giddiness, headache, nausea, vomiting, sweating, thirst, palpitations and difficulty in urinating, along with restlessness and insomnia, while some people may experience those symptoms with the usual therapeutic dosage.

I concluded that at the time of the incident, given the quantity of drugs found, it was very unlikely that they were all for Harvey's personal use. This was further supported by the fact that the tablets and blister-seal packets had been removed from their cardboard packaging. I had clearly understated the situation.

Harvey was subsequently charged with possessing a precursor for use in the manufacture/production of a prohibited drug, although he was granted conditional bail and the matter put-over to the following year, where it was to go before Dubbo Local Court on 8 February 2006. After much toing and froing with the defence counsel, the matter was then put-over for a hearing, which was subsequently set down for 26 and 27 June 2006.

I was informed that the defence still wanted to cross-examine me regarding the statement I'd prepared, and so a flight and accommodation were booked and I packed an overnight bag, ready to fly to Dubbo. I was on my way.

However, at the metaphoric last minute, I was informed that my 43-page statement had been accepted and handed to the court. I was no longer required to attend the session. Given the lead-up to the hearing, the turn of events was quite unusual, but that's life.

I didn't find out about the outcome of the matter, but section 10 of the *Drug Misuse and Trafficking Act 1985* (NSW) simply states that a person who has a prohibited drug in his or her possession is guilty of an offence, and the maximum penalty for the offence of possessing a prohibited drug is a fine of $5500 and/or two years imprisonment.

Harvey's $3000 would have made a good deposit.

Good Coke, Good Dope: Bad Combination

'Happiness lies within one's self,
and the way to dig it out is cocaine.'
— *Aleister Crowley,* **Diary of a Drug Fiend**

Cocaine is a potent stimulant drug found in the leaves of the coca bush (*Erythroxylon coca*) in amounts ranging from 0.25 to 2 per cent by weight. The shrub is native to the Andean highlands of South America and the leaves have been chewed by Peruvian natives since very ancient times to ward off hunger and weariness caused by the altitude and thirst.

It was first extracted and purified in 1855 by German chemist, Friedrich Gaedcke, and since then the drug has been used in medicine as a local anaesthetic (particularly in dentistry and ophthalmological procedures). Even Sigmund Freud, the noted Austrian neurologist and founder of psychoanalysis, touted the virtues of the drug as a therapeutic tonic in his 1884 paper 'Über Coca', in which he said that cocaine could cure depression and sexual impotence.

Unfortunately, the drug's addictive properties were not recognised until 1925, when the Geneva Convention decided that it had to become a controlled drug. Since then, it's been increasingly used by drug abusers for its euphoric and stimulatory properties, and has become a very profitable business for drug lords and smugglers. Cocaine has many street names, such as 'nose candy' (due to one of the methods of ingestion), 'snow', 'toot', 'white lady' and 'coke'. It's most commonly taken intranasally ('snorting' the powder), but it can be injected, and as a freebase and in the form of crack cocaine, it can be smoked.

Immediately after smoking or intravenous injection, the cocaine user experiences an intense sensation, called a rush or flash, which only lasts a few minutes, but has been described as very pleasurable. Oral or intranasal use produces euphoria – a high – but not a rush.

Unlike cocaine, heroin is a potent central nervous system depressant drug that is semi-synthetic, meaning that the drug, while derived from natural sources, is subsequently chemically modified. Heroin, chemically known as diacetylmorphine or diamorphine, as the name suggests, is derived from morphine, one of the major alkaloids present in the latex of the opium poppy (*Papaver somniferum*). It was first synthesised by C.R. Alder Wright in 1874 by reacting two acetyl groups (using acetic acid, a component of vinegar) to morphine. Curiously, Wright's synthesis of diamorphine didn't lead to any further developments until 1897, when the drug was re-synthesised by Felix Hoffman, who was working at the Bayer pharmaceutical company in Elberfeld, Germany. The drug was subsequently commercialised under the trade name heroin, based on the German heroisch, which means 'heroic'. It was (is) an analgesic with about twice the potency of morphine.

From 1898 to 1910, diamorphine was marketed by Bayer under the trademark heroin and was used for pain relief and as a cough suppressant. After the defeat of Germany in World War I, the trademark rights were lost under the 1919 Treaty of Versailles.

By 1925, the powerful addictive properties of diamorphine were recognised and the health committee of the League of Nations had the drug banned. It's now a scheduled (prohibited) drug in many countries, including Australia.

However, due to the intense euphoria it produces, that hasn't stopped the widespread use of heroin as a recreational drug, and because tolerance to it develops quickly, ever increasing doses are needed to achieve the same effects.

Heroin addicts can become quite tolerant to large amounts of morphine, but even they can, and do, die from overdoses. Generally, however, the toxic dose of morphine for a non-addicted person is somewhere in the region of 60 milligrams, and serious symptoms are usually experienced after doses of 100 milligrams. The outlook becomes less favourable as the dosage increases, and doses above 250 milligrams carry a serious prognosis, with death occurring as a result of marked respiratory depression and consequent anoxia (total lack of oxygen).

★

Over the years, I've received many cases where people have overdosed on either cocaine or heroin, and in some cases they've consumed alcohol as well, thus contributing to the toxicity of the drug, with a fatal outcome. I can only think of a few cases over my career where both cocaine and heroin were consumed at the same time, along with alcohol, but the story that follows is one of those.

Stuart Bradley Lovell was born in Geelong, Victoria on 30 April 1981. He was a bit of a rover and lived in a number of different locations around Australia, including Broome, Perth, Geelong and Brisbane, before finally settling in Darwin. He was a likeable, happy, easygoing person who avoided confrontation, but he dabbled in marijuana (cannabis) and ecstasy as a recreational user before graduating later to the more expensive hard stuff — heroin and cocaine.

In early February 2008, he began work as a consultant with Kelly Services (Australia) Ltd, a recruitment company with a number of offices throughout Australia. As part of the recruitment process, new consultants were required to attend a training session, which was held in Sydney, New South Wales. Lovell was a keen participant in the training course; perhaps not surprisingly, as out of the six course participants, he was the only male. On Tuesday 19 February, he boarded a flight from Darwin to Brisbane and then took a connecting flight to Sydney, where he caught a cab from the airport and checked into the Ibis Hotel in Pitt Street, at the southern end of the Sydney CBD, where he had a reservation.

The intensive training course was scheduled for two days, concluding on Thursday the 21st, when it was time to 'chill out' and relax. Along with several course participants, Lovell went off to a hotel in The Rocks to have a few drinks before returning to the Ibis. The Rocks is a popular tourist precinct located on the southern shore of Sydney Harbour, not far from Circular Quay.

Back at the Ibis, he changed his clothing and then met up with a fellow course participant, Jackalene 'Jackie' Ellis in the hotel foyer. She was also staying at the hotel. They caught a taxi to the Four Seasons Hotel at The Rocks and met Jayne Ormerod at 8 pm, outside the hotel.

They walked around Circular Quay and past the Museum of Contemporary Art, before having dinner and drinks at the Lowenbrau bar/restaurant in The Rocks. While at the Lowenbrau, Stuart drank about a litre of German beer, having one during dinner and another later. Clearly a thirsty fellow. During the course of the dinner, he received several calls on his mobile phone, prompting Jayne to turn to him and ask what he was doing. Stuart looked at Jackie and they both laughed. Jackie said, 'He's under the thumb,' and explained that his girlfriend in Darwin was constantly calling him because she was concerned he was the only male on the course.

They left the Lowenbrau bar at about 10.30 pm and went to the Argyle Hotel next door, by which time Stuart was very affected by the alcohol he'd consumed, and after having further drinks of gin and cranberry juice, he was described as 'pretty drunk', if one can call being drunk pretty. Following further drinks, the trio caught a taxi to Kings Cross, where they parted company, with Stuart Lovell saying, 'I'm just going across the road to a strip joint.' In the meantime, for some inexplicable reason, Jackie decided she wanted to get a tattoo, and the two young women went into a nearby tattoo parlour. While Jackie was getting her tattoo, Jayne became concerned about Stuart, as he wasn't from Sydney, and sent him a text message. Stuart replied and discovered the young women were only a short distance away. Jayne then saw him and waved.

But Stuart was not himself, appearing to be 'drunk and kind of twitchy', and he told Jayne and Jackie that he was waiting for a girl and would catch up with them the following day.

With that, they bid their farewells and the young women headed off to their hotels. That was the last time Stuart Lovell was seen by his female colleagues.

The following morning, Jackie sent Stuart a text at 6.45 am. Are you awake, are we meeting for breakfast or shall I meet you in the lobby?

She received a reply soon after.

No, I'm tired, still in bed. Met a lady last night. I'll catch you later. I'll call you in half an hour.

Jackie responded: Have fun sleeping in, don't forget to call Jayne and Gareth (coordinators of the training course) to let them know. See you later.

Jayne also phoned Stuart and left a message on his phone, asking him to call back. At about 10.30 am, after not getting a reply, she rang the Ibis Hotel and asked someone to check on him. While waiting on the line, the receptionist told her he was sleeping.

Time ticked by and midday came around. Check-out time had been at 11 am, so the receptionist asked the housekeeping supervisor to check on the room, as the occupant still hadn't left. The supervisor knocked twice on the door and called out, 'Housekeeping, can I come in?'

After getting no response, she entered the room and was confronted with an awful sight. Stuart Lovell was lying on his back, on the floor, in between a bed and a desk. A pinkish-red foam was emerging from his nostrils, and a pillow, which had some blood on it, had been placed under his head. There were two small sealed bags nearby, one on the table and the other on the floor. A spoon containing a white residue lay alongside the body, together with an empty needle packet. The room was very messy and untidy with clothing on the floor and various personal items spread on the table. It appeared to have been a busy and active, if fatal, night. Jayne Ormerod's concerns for Stuart had been well-founded.

In extreme shock, the housekeeper, fearing the worst, quickly left the room and called out to a fellow employee, who took a quick look and said, 'He's just drunk and has passed out.'

Unfortunately, the situation was far more serious and complicated.

Due to the circumstances, the assistant hotel manager and housekeeping manager (it's apparently standard practice that two people enter a room together if there is a problem) were now very concerned as to why the occupant of the room hadn't checked out of the hotel as previously arranged. They knocked twice on the room door and received no response, so they opened the door and watched Lovell for a short time, but didn't see him breathing. Realising that he was most likely dead, an ambulance was called. On arrival, the paramedics confirmed their fears, and a doctor later issued a death certificate.

A night of celebration had ended in a tragedy – and Stuart was only 26 years old.

His body arrived in a sealed body bag at the Glebe Department of Forensic Medicine on that Friday afternoon of 22 February. The post-mortem was carried out by Dr Istvan Szentmariay at 9 am on the morning of 25 February. A number of tattoos were observed on his body, but more importantly, there were recent intravenous (IV) track marks on his right elbow, a recent underlying subcutaneous haemorrhage and his lungs were congested. It looked like another drug overdose. That was borne out by the subsequent toxicology report, which revealed that a blood sample taken from Lovell's body at the post-mortem was found to contain morphine 0.24 milligrams per litre, codeine 0.07 milligrams per litre (in this case a probable metabolite of a large dose of morphine), cocaine 0.53 milligrams per litre, benzoylecgonine 0.90 milligrams per litre (a metabolite of cocaine) and alcohol 0.101 grams per decilitre (100 millilitres) of blood or 0.101%.

A very toxic and fatal mix.

Additionally, there was a large quantity of morphine in his bile, indicating either a very large injection of an opiate or, more likely, a number of injections over time, resulting in a build-up of the drug in the fluid. The presence of monoacetylmorphine in his urine indicated that the morphine was most likely derived from heroin use. Further tests later showed that to be the case.

I concluded that the levels of cocaine and morphine, together with a mid-range alcohol concentration in Stuart Bradley Lovell's blood was consistent with an overdosage of these drugs, resulting in his death.

The direct cause of his death was subsequently described as, 'mixed opiate and cocaine toxicity'. A simple explanation for a more complicated situation.

The white powders and residue in the spoon that were found in Lovell's room were analysed and found to contain cocaine, diacetylmorphine (heroin), monoacetylmorphine (a breakdown product of heroin) and acetylcodeine (an impurity often found in street-grade heroin). It appeared that the young man had taken a mixture of cocaine and street-grade heroin. That's a classic drug combination known as a speed ball, although mixing any stimulant and depressant can be described as speed balling. For example, mixing Xanax (alprazolam) with methylamphetamine (meth).

But why speed ball when you can get a high from either drug?

The answer lies in the fact that heroin is a central nervous system depressant drug while cocaine is a stimulant, and by mixing the two drugs, users experience the intense rush of cocaine, followed by the sedating effects of heroin. Also, because cocaine has a short-lived high, adding heroin to the mix helps with the eventual crash when the effects of the cocaine wear off. Effectively, speed balling results in an overwhelming and pleasurable high. Users typically inject that drug combination several times in a night.

The large quantity of morphine in Stuart's bile indicated that that was the most probable scenario.

His girl for the night had obviously come well-equipped with her recreational drugs, but in addition to the toxic mix, Lovell had also consumed a large amount of alcohol earlier in the evening.

Ibis Hotel CCTV footage from Thursday 21 February showed Stuart Lovell carrying his black and orange backpack and going to his room at about 6.30 pm. He was seen to leave the hotel at approximately 6.40 pm. Further CCTV footage from Friday 22 February showed him returning the Ibis Hotel at about 3.30 am with an unknown woman. She was seen leaving from the direction of his room at about 8 am.

She was carrying a white plastic bag and a bulging orange and black backpack on her back.

A number of checks were made on Lovell's mobile phone, and they indicated he'd contacted a person living in Tempe. Further investigations revealed the mystery woman's identity through a DNA profile that was lifted from a cigarette butt found in Lovell's room. The woman (who cannot be identified) was known to police and was not only addicted to illicit drugs, in particular cocaine and heroin, but also had a lengthy history of stealing, assault, drug usage and professing her love of cocaine. She was a frequent visitor to Kings Cross, which was where Stuart had met her and organised for her to come back to his hotel room. It was there that he'd been introduced to a speed ball injection, and most likely relied on the assistance of the girl to inject the cocktail of cocaine and heroin. It was also likely that as he succumbed to the deadly mix of drugs and alcohol, the girl placed a pillow under his head before leaving the room with some of his possessions in the orange and black backpack.

This case is reminiscent of the death of a talented soccer coach, Ian 'Iggy' Avenel Gray, who died in similar circumstances from a mixture of drugs which consisted of stimulants (methylamphetamine, cocaine, phentermine) and the depressant heroin. The shot of heroin had been administered by an escort he'd engaged for the evening, and when his body was discovered, the same ominous foam as was observed with Stuart Lovell was seen emerging from his nostrils.

That is a typical diagnostic from a 'speed balling' overdose. Unfortunately, there have been a number of celebrities that have met their end that way, including River Phoenix, who was only 23 years old, John Belushi (aged 33), Brent Mydland (aged 37) and a number of others only recorded in morgue documents. Apparently, even King George V of England succumbed to the drug mixture. He was chronically ill from a lung disease and needed relief from the complaint, so his personal physician, Lord Dawson, allegedly gave him a mixed dose of cocaine and morphine.

Which just goes to show that even in the 1930s, 'speed balling' was a problem.

Stuart Lovell's remains were returned to his birthplace in Geelong, Victoria to be buried with his father, Daryl Lovell, who had passed away 17 years earlier. Unlike a number of cases I've had in the past, his family had closure, but far too many young people remain lost and unaccounted for.

There's the true tragedy.

Affairs of the Heart and Poison

'If you drink from a bottle marked 'poison',
you are bound to suffer.'
– Lewis Carroll

The vast majority of poisoning cases with which I was involved and provided expert advice/evidence for at local, district and supreme court levels dealt mostly with the more common drugs. For example, stimulants such as MDMA (ecstasy), methamphetamine, amphetamine, ephedrine, phentermine, and central nervous system depressants such as morphine, heroin, benzodiazepines (diazepam, oxazepam etc.), cannabis, methadone and, of course, alcohol. However, from time to time, unusual poisons appeared in my casework. One such case involved a pesticide rather than drugs.

★

Back in 2001, a couple in a small country town were going through some marital difficulties, and the bored farmer's wife embarked on a number of affairs. What had started out as a passionate romance with her 'wild man' soon soured as the dreary reality of marital duties and farm life set in. But country towns being what they are, word soon reached her husband, and when he discovered her most recent liaison, he decided that enough was enough and plotted to murder her.

Being a farmer, he'd had occasion to use Phosdrin to kill foxes that had threatened his livestock, and still had plenty of it in one of his sheds. He determined it would be ideal for what he had in mind.

The only problem was how to administer it without his wife noticing. Fortunately for the farmer, she was into natural therapy products, a form of homeopathy, and took colloidal silver (believed to be a naturopathic treatment for asthma) every day, so on the morning of 20 May, the farmer added half a mil (millilitre) of Phosdrin to her colloidal silver and waited for the inevitable.

However, things didn't go according to plan. His wife took one sip of the colloidal silver and was immediately alerted to its foul and different taste. She spat out what was in her mouth and rinsed with cold water, but couldn't avoid swallowing a small amount. Later on, she felt woozy, was unable to focus properly, was shaking badly, had no control over her bowels and threw up violently over the toilet floor. Somehow, she managed to call for an ambulance. When it arrived, she was sitting in a chair, sobbing. The paramedics asked her what had happened, to which she replied, 'My husband's poisoned me.' She was rushed to hospital, where she recovered, having more or less saved her own life through her prompt actions of spitting and rinsing and subsequent involuntary vomiting.

The treating doctor took a blood sample, which was examined for the presence of mevinphos (Phosdrin), but none was detected. However, a search of the farm turned up a bottle of red liquid marked Phosdrin, which contained mevinphos, as did the colloidal silver medication. Mevinphos was also detected in a drinking glass and in the vomit-stained towel taken from the toilet.

No matter how it's administered, mevinphos is a highly toxic organophosphorus insecticide. It affects the central nervous system and the eyes, and its action is direct and quick. Toxic effects include nausea, vomiting, diarrhoea, abdominal cramps, headache, dizziness, blurred vision, salivation, sweating and confusion, and they can appear within 15 minutes to two hours after exposure. It was developed from a nerve gas program during the Second World War, and along with its close cousins (various chemical analogues) is designed to kill – and kill very effectively.

The husband was initially charged with attempted murder, but when the matter went to trial, some legal wrangling saw the charge reduced to administering poison with intent to injure. However, in an unbelievable turn of events, the wife became the defence's star witness by changing her evidence, or as the police termed it, she 'did a backflip in the witness box'.

This is part of what she said, 'I felt that he only did it to frighten me. He could probably have cut my throat, or he could have given me a whole heap, and given me a cup of tea. Phosdrin works within three seconds.' (Note: Not even deadly cyanide works that fast.)

I wasn't called to give expert testimony and let the court know just how close to death the farmer's wife had come, but when I spoke to the Department of Public Prosecutions and asked what sentence would be appropriate for an offence of that nature, they indicated at least a period of penal servitude.

In the event, the farmer was given just 250 hours of community service. Not bad for attempted murder – which most likely could have succeeded.

The Case of the One-Armed Would-Be Rapist

'First you take a drink, then the drink takes a drink,
then the drink takes you.'
– F. Scott Fitzgerald

Because of its easy availability, alcohol is the drug most commonly associated with sexual assault cases. It's rapidly absorbed into the bloodstream after ingestion and distributes throughout the entire body, including, most importantly, the central nervous system (CNS), where its depressant effects are the most profound. In drug-facilitated sexual assault cases, the victims quite often consume the alcohol voluntarily, particularly when the perpetrator provides the alcoholic beverage in copious quantities to the potential victim. Alcohol decreases inhibitions, impairs perception and may cause loss of consciousness and/or amnesia, especially when other CNS drugs, such as diazepam, are used as well.

★

On the cool evening of 12 July 2006, Sandra Clooney met up with Ken Grose for a social drink at the Five Dock Hotel. Ken had had a hard life, having lost an arm in an industrial accident, and he was keen to get back on the social scene. The couple chatted away quite amicably, and throughout the evening, Ken kept Sandra well supplied with drinks, ranging from VBs to Sambuca (an anise-flavoured liqueur). Perhaps unsurprisingly, Sandra started to be affected by the alcohol, becoming quite light-headed as well as exhibiting some more obvious outward signs such as uttering the occasional slurred word and becoming more voluble. Ken wasn't slow in noticing the deterioration and thought it was going to be his lucky night. The real giveaway was when Sandra said, 'Go … osh, I feel quite pissed, Ken.'

Being nothing if not a gentleman, Ken went up to the bar and ordered more drinks, saying to the staff, 'I'm going to get a root [have sex] tonight.'

He was a subtle bloke!

The extra drinks weren't really necessary, given what Ken Grose had in mind, because by the time he got back to the table, he could see Sandra was well under the weather and quite incapable of getting herself home. Leaving the drinks, he took her outside and she got into his vehicle, thinking that Ken was going to drive her home. However, he had another idea in mind. As he drove, Sandra dozed off. She was obviously far gone and Ken had drunk enough to be emboldened to act out his fantasy.

He pulled over, stopped his motor vehicle, opened the door and dragged Sandra out, both of them spilling into the gutter alongside the road. Sandra didn't stir, so he undid her jeans and pulled both them and her panties down before unzipping the fly of his pants.

Unfortunately for Ken, things were not about to go to plan, and a police officer on his way back to the station after dealing with another matter at the nearby Western Suburbs Soccer Club noticed them. He went back to the club and asked the manager and doorman of the club to accompany him as witnesses. When they returned, Sandra was lying face down on the roadway, her jeans and panties down to her knees, with Ken on top of her, moving his pelvis slowly up and down over her exposed bottom.

'Hey, what's going on here?' the officer asked.

Ken stood up, revealing the fly of his pants was undone. Sandra, being unconscious, remained where she was.

A comatose Sandra was placed in the police car and driven to the hospital, while Ken was taken to the police station and charged with attempted sexual assault. When Sandra regained consciousness, she didn't have a clue where she was and was totally unaware of what had happened to her.

She was subjected to testing, involving a sexual assault investigation kit (SAIK), in which blood and urine samples were taken. The samples were then forwarded to an accredited laboratory for analysis.

A blood sample taken the following day, at 12 pm, 10 hours after Sandra and Ken had been taken in by the police, was found to contain ecstasy or 3, 4-methylenedioxymethylamphetamine (MDMA) 0.10 milligrams per litre, pseudoephedrine 0.05 milligrams per litre (possibly, an impurity in the MDMA preparation), diazepam less than 0.1 milligrams per litre, nordiazepam less than 0.1 milligrams per litre, and more significantly, alcohol 0.125 grams per 100 millilitres (decilitre) of blood. The diazepam and nordiazapam readings indicated that a drug such as Valium had been taken sometime earlier.

When asked what her blood alcohol level would have been at 2 am, about the time Sandra and Ken were caught in the act, I said that the lowest possible reading would have been 0.225 grams per decilitre of blood and the highest reading 0.375 grams, with a more probable reading of 0.325 grams. While Sandra was a seasoned drinker of alcohol (and she apparently had a problem in that area), they were very high readings, which alone would have accounted for her condition (as observed by witnesses and police) before even taking the other drugs detected in her blood into account. Consequently, her ability to ward off Ken's unwanted sexual advances were severely compromised.

The matter ended up in court, where the magistrate found that the prosecution had failed to produce enough evidence that Ken had attempted to rape Sandra, as penile penetration appeared not to have occurred. Ken was cleared and the case was dismissed.

As one wag was overheard saying on leaving the court, 'Yeah, he was armless but not 'armless!'

I could not disagree.

A 'Meth'-Fuelled Madness with a Shocking End

'I wanted to meet the monster.
Why go down if you can go up?'
– Ellen Hopkins, Crank

Wagga, or more accurately Wagga Wagga, is a major regional city in the Riverina region of New South Wales. The original inhabitants of the region were the Wiradjuri people, and the term derived from their language apparently means 'crow', when repeated, it means 'many', or essentially 'many crows'. Wagga is a delightful country town that straddles the Murrumbidgee River, which is fed by the melt waters from the Snowy Mountains. It's situated almost midway between Sydney and Melbourne and in the 2014 census, the urban centre of Wagga was recorded as having a population of 62,799. It is one of the largest inland towns in New South Wales.

It was in this setting that another country road tragedy occurred. But this one was quite unique: while drugs were involved, the ending for the driver was quite shocking, in more ways than one, and most unexpected.

★

On a pleasant Sunday afternoon on 23 March 2014, Aaron Anthony Crain was observed to be speeding down Copland Street, Wagga Wagga. Unfortunately for him, his driving manner was detected by Wagga highway police who subsequently pulled him over and he was routinely breath tested. He only registered low range alcohol. When he was told that he was positive for alcohol, his whole demeanour changed. He suddenly became very agitated and leaped out of the car exclaiming, 'What can do I do, what can I do? I'm just gunna kill myself!'

It was an extraordinary overreaction.

With that, he bolted to a nearby 'A Frame' powerline transmission tower at the intersection of Tasman Road and Copland Street in Wagga Wagga and climbed the tower with police officers in hot pursuit. But to no avail.

Aaron had succeeded in climbing to the first transmission line of the tower when suddenly a current of high-voltage electricity was observed to arc from the second transmission line into his body causing him to fall about 30 metres to the ground.

Ambulance officers were called to the scene, but it soon became obvious that no signs of life were present and so, no resuscitative efforts were initiated.

It was quite literally, a truly shocking end for a young man only 30 years old.

Aaron Crain's body was taken to the Department of Forensic Medicine, Sydney where a post-mortem was carried out by Dr Kendall Bailey at 9.30 am on 25 March 2014.

The post-mortem showed that Aaron Crain had received traumatic injuries to his head along with fractures to his upper and lower limbs and his chest wall. No doubt due to the fall from the tower.

In addition, there were extensive electrical injuries over his body and singed clothing consistent with high-voltage electrocution. These were expected, given the circumstances of his death.

The coroner found that the direct cause of death was due to multiple blunt-force injuries along with high-voltage electrical injuries.

The subsequent toxicology report of the blood samples taken from

Aaron Crain at the post-mortem stated that his blood contained alcohol 0.049 grams per decilitre (0.049%) – just under the legal limit, delta-9-THC acid less than 0.010 milligrams per litre (indicating he had smoked cannabis sometime earlier) and more importantly, methylamphetamine ('meth') 0.22 milligrams per litre.

The main player which led to this tragedy was the stimulant, methylamphetamine.

The therapeutic range for it (methamphetamine or just meth) in blood is 0.01 to 0.05 mg/L. Within that range, the drug has an appealing combination of mild to moderate central nervous system stimulating effects. However, levels well above that range (depending upon usage and tolerance) can result in increased wakefulness, increased physical activity, decreased appetite, increased respiration and hyperthermia. But worse, the drug can impair a user's faculties by altering perceptions and judgement and increase aggressive or risk-taking behaviour. And if the levels are high enough, the drug may also produce hallucinations.

Aaron Crain's blood level of methylamphetamine was just over four times the top end of the therapeutic range. It had clearly affected his behaviour.

However, in this instance he sought not to taken another's life (as described in an earlier story) but his own.

'Meth' can be a monster in many ways.

A Case of Misdiagnosis: An Arsenic Poisoning?

'The fact that your patient gets well, does not prove
that your diagnosis was correct.'
– Samuel J. Meltz

Arsenic has been used in medicines, as a pigment, a pesticide – and as a poison to commit murder. The element occurs widely throughout the environment in many minerals, usually in conjunction with sulphur and various metals such as lead, zinc, iron and copper. Arsenic is one of the most toxic of the naturally occurring elements in nature. It has more effects on health than any other toxicant and is known to cause cancer of the skin, bladder, lungs, kidney and liver. The final result of chronic arsenic poisoning is coma and death.

Symptoms of arsenic poisoning occur with headaches, confusion, stomach cramps and diarrhoea. As the poisoning progresses, convulsions and changes in fingernail pigmentation called leukonychia striata or Mees' lines may occur. When the poisoning becomes acute, the symptoms intensify including severe diarrhoea, vomiting, cramping muscles, hair loss and more convulsions.

Arsenic poisoning often occurs from contaminated groundwater that contains high levels of arsenic and has been associated with increased deaths from cardiovascular disease. Environmental exposures from contaminated drinking water and airborne workplace exposures have been the main focus of various investigations. By contrast, the toxicological significance of naturally occurring arsenic in foods has received relatively less attention. The largest quantity of dietary arsenic comes from saltwater fin-fish and seafood such as crustaceans, prawns and lobsters, the latter of which can contain up to 22 milligrams per kilogram of tissue, most of which is organically bound.

★

It was a relatively quiet morning in the office when I received an enquiry from a police officer who was investigating a poisoning incident. His client (the victim 'Mr Jones') had attended Miranda Police Station with his solicitor and said that he believed his wife was trying to poison him. Mr Jones explained that in September 2009, he became sick and started suffering from chronic diarrhoea. This continued until he separated from his wife in July 2010. He said it took about three weeks for the symptoms to slowly go away. Then about three to four weeks later Mr Jones received a call from his ex-wife's best friend. During the conversation the friend revealed that the ex-wife had been poisoning him for some time. This supposedly, explained the ongoing sickness he was experiencing. Arsenic was suspected.

Mr Jones subsequently went to his local doctor who, on hearing his patient's symptoms, decided to have his patient's urine tested. It returned a positive result for arsenic. Maybe his fears were well-founded.

I suggested that a blood sample should be taken, along with a sample of hair taken from the nape of the neck, and fingernail clippings. In the hair arsenic becomes chemically bonded to the sulphur atoms in the keratin molecules from which hair is made. Hair is a wonderful 'timeline' to determine chronic ingestion of various substances that the body has been exposed to, including arsenic. Unfortunately, the alleged victim had very short hair, so we had to settle for the nail clippings and a blood sample.

The latter sample only provided a 'snapshot' of the toxin levels. While the nail clippings were sampled to determine chronic exposure, as a further check a urine sample was also taken and submitted for analysis.

Mr Jones' fingernails were examined and the expected Mees' lines were inconclusive. The urine sample once again returned a positive result for arsenic of 125 micrograms per litre. This was high, though not a toxic result, given the usual base level is about 50 micrograms per litre or less. However, the blood and nail clippings results were negative for arsenic.

What was going on?

It appeared that the arsenic was most likely from a dietary source and not necessarily a case of deliberate poisoning. Mr Jones was questioned about his diet and his food preferences. He admitted he 'loved seafood' in particular, prawns, shellfish and lobster.

A prawn species he particularly enjoyed was the tiger prawn (*Penaeus esculentus*) and he had a sumptuous meal of these crustaceans only two days earlier at the local bowling club. Prawn heads tend to concentrate most of the heavy metals. This is due to the fact that the head contains the hepatopancreas, an organ known to be an important metal storage site in decapod crustaceans. The tail flesh – and this is the tissue most people eat – had the lowest concentrations of all metals except mercury – and arsenic.

This looked like an explanation for the elevated levels of arsenic detected in Mr Jones' urine and, possibly, some of his symptoms. The consumption of seafood, crustaceans in particular, within two to three days of testing can increase total urine arsenic concentrations. Unfortunately, few clinicians are aware of this fact and often misinterpret elevated results. This case proved to be no exception, producing an unnecessary referral, further testing and a very anxious client.

Hopefully, this was not the only reason that led to his separation from his wife!

Drugs and Driving:
A Roadside Tragedy

'There's a killer on the road.
His [her] brain is swerving like a toad.'
– Jim Morrison 'Riders on the Storm'

There are many things happening around you when you drive. It is necessary to be totally focused so that in a split-second, when a potentially life-saving decision needs to be made, you're ready to react. Whether it be to hit the brake to avoid hitting a thoughtless pedestrian on a mobile phone or to take evasive action to avoid a collision with another road user. Driving is a very complex task.

However, drugs can greatly affect your ability to react and so increase the chances of an accident. Stimulants such as amphetamines, can cause a driver to become overconfident and aggressive, and take unnecessary risks. While sedatives such as diazepam and cannabis can cause a driver to become sleepy and inattentive, and either drift off the road or into other traffic. Both scenarios have the potential to cause serious accidents. Not a good result.

In all my years working as a forensic toxicologist, I have never been able to understand why people take drugs (both illicit and licit) – and drive. The highway is challengingly enough without 'demons' in your head!

★

It was approaching mid-morning on a warm Christmas Day in 2009, when Ms Brodie Donegan decided to take a short walk to stretch her legs outside an Ourimbah property on the Central Coast, New South Wales, that she shared with her partner, Nick Ball. Brody was 28 years old and she and her partner were looking forward to the birth of a daughter. So much so, Brodie then 32-weeks pregnant, and Nick had already named their unborn daughter Zoe (Greek for 'life').

Only a couple of months to go before the joyous occasion!

Meanwhile, Ms Justine Hampson, 40, was loading her six-year-old child into her van. Unfortunately, the evening previously Ms Hampson who had a number of health issues, had consumed a number of Valium tablets and a dose of Xanax, along with a dose of methadone earlier that morning.

No doubt she was feeling a bit under the weather as she made the fateful decision to drive her vehicle to Ourimbah. As Ms Hampson drove along the highway, she passed another vehicle and then began drifting off the road, not realising her vehicle was headed straight towards Ms Donegan.

There was no time for her to jump out of the way of the careering vehicle.

There was a sickening thump as the van slammed into the body of the pregnant young woman. At about 10.30 am, alerted to the ensuing awful commotion, neighbours called police who quickly arrived at the scene, closely followed by an ambulance. On examination by paramedics, they soon realised that Ms Donegan was in a very bad way, having suffered terrible injuries which included a shattered pelvis, thigh, lower spine and a damaged foot. Clearly, given her injuries and advanced pregnancy, she wouldn't be able to handle to the road trip to Sydney and she was airlifted by helicopter to Royal North Shore Hospital (RNSH) where she underwent an emergency caesarean. Sadly, despite the best efforts of the surgeons at RNSH, her daughter Zoe was stillborn.

As the helicopter had left for RNSH with the seriously injured patient, police turned their attention to Ms Hampson and as per protocol she was subjected to a breath test. The test was negative for alcohol. However, when spoken to by police she was observed to be cooperative and sedated, while her eyes were glazed and speech slow. Her movements overall were sluggish.

Police were convinced Ms Hampson was under the influence of drugs, and a medical officer was summoned and blood and urine samples were taken from for subsequent analysis and testing.

The analyst's report (carried out by the Division of Analytical Laboratories, Lidcombe, New South Wales) showed that at 1.30 pm on 25 December 2009, Ms Hampson had the following levels of drugs in her blood: diazepam 1.5 milligrams per litre and its metabolites; nordiazepam 0.27 milligrams per litre, oxazepam 0.02 milligrams and temazepam 0.13 milligrams per litre, alprazolam 0.02 milligrams per litre, along with methadone 0.23 milligrams per litre. Moclobemide was detected in her urine sample.

While the level of diazepam (and its respective active metabolites) was significant, along with the presence of alprazolam, and with the additive effects from methadone. I opined that it was the drug combination that severely affected her driving ability leading to the tragic outcome. All of these drugs, while legal, have sedative effects and thereby affect driving ability.

To elaborate, diazepam is a benzodiazepine-type sedative that is available under the trade names Valium and Ducene, which is used in the short-term relief of anxiety symptoms. Its metabolites (essentially break-down products) namely, nordiazepam, oxazepam and temazepam are drugs in their own right and exert sedative effects on the consumer.

Alprazolam is also a benzodiazepine-type sedative from the same drug class, which is available under several trade names including Xanax, which is used in the short-term relief of depression and panic disorder.

Methadone, another drug detected in her system, is a narcotic analgesic that is generally used as a substitute for heroin in those suffering from addiction. Most folk, on a stabilised program, would not be affected by the drug and could possibly drive without serious impairment of their abilities. But, and this is an important but, significant impairment will occur if methadone is used with other central nervous system depressant drugs such as diazepam and alprazolam.

Ms Hampson had both, along with methadone.

Further, moclobemide was also detected in her urine. This was yet another antidepressant drug Ms Hampson was taking, which is known under the various trade names as Arima and Aurorix.

All of these drugs individually, could have impaired Ms Hampson's ability to drive. But, in combination, it was a drug cocktail mixture for disaster and certainly, when it came to any complex task, such as driving.

And sadly, that was the outcome.

Ms Hampson was convicted of two charges namely, dangerous driving and causing grievous bodily harm. The Department of Public Prosecutions decided there was sufficient grounds for the matter to go to trial.

In the meantime, Ms Donegan had to undergo seven months of painful rehabilitation to repair her shattered pelvis, lower spine and leg. It was a very dark period of Brodie Donegan's life. One that should never have happened.

On 14 July 2010, Justine Hampson faced Wyong Local Court for the first time to answer the charges. No doubt, Ms Donegan was looking forward to finalising the matter. Unfortunately, it wasn't to be so, and the prosecutor told the court that the officer-in-charge hadn't completed his evidence saying, 'I've spoken to the officer in charge, most of the brief has been completed. The medical evidence has not been received.'

Outside the court, Ms Donegan said that police had only recently asked her consent to release her medical records. 'It's stupid,' she complained, 'You would think they would have everything ready, especially since I've been the one riding them all this time.'

Unfortunately, this sad case was to be further delayed due to various administrative problems, resulting in months of adjournments. Further, to add to her frustration, Ms Donegan learned that police had not suspended Ms Hampson's driver licence. This is standard procedure when blood tests return a positive test for controlled substances. However, this 'hiccup' was probably due to the fact that the drugs detected in Ms Hampson's system were legal – not controlled substances such as cannabis, methamphetamine, MDMA and heroin. And despite some media reports, she was not 'high' on a cocktail of prescription drugs and alcohol. No alcohol was detected in Ms Hampson's blood sample.

Then, to further complicate matters, there was a large backlog of driving under the influence drug matters due to the lack of staff both at the DAL laboratory and the CFMU.

But on a more cheery note, Brodie Donegan being a very resilient young woman and despite her injuries, revealed she was again pregnant at 28 weeks with another child. Due to her severe injuries, she was understandably nervous about a possible complicated birth outcome.

Mr Ball commented, 'It's not going to be the best time of year for us right now but it's good to get some closure.'

Eventually, on 30 March 2011 the matter went before Judge Roy Ellis at the Gosford District Court for sentencing.

It had been some 15 agonising months since Brodie Donegan was hit by a van on Christmas Day 2009, resulting in the loss of her unborn baby girl.

But the main thing that would have dominated her thoughts that day was to hear an apology from the driver for the tragedy. In court, Justine Hampson did the unexpected and decent thing, she pleaded both guilty and apologised to Ms Donegan.

The injured mother was surprised and accepted it, adding it meant a lot to her.

Ms Hampson, then 41 years old, sobbed as Ms Donegan wept while reading her victim impact statement about her short walk that severely injured her body and claimed the life of her second daughter Zoe when Ms Donegan was 32 weeks pregnant.

Nevertheless, Judge Roy Ellis found her guilty of dangerous driving causing grievous bodily harm to Ms Donegan and driving under the influence of prescribed drugs. Ms Hampson was subsequently sentenced to nine months jail.

However, the sentence could have been good deal longer – up to two years. Judge Ellis took into consideration the impact of a jail sentence on Ms Hampson's two children, who included a special needs intellectually and physically handicapped teenage son. He recognised her remorse was genuine and factored in her mental health issues. In addition, Justine Hampson had had a difficult life described as 'very problematic', which included being sexually abused as a child, the early deaths of both parents and a dubious relationship with a heroin addict which in turn, led to her becoming a heroin addict.

It was truly a tragic tale of two mothers.

Murder in the Blue Mountains? The Death of Margaret Hills

'Life itself is but the shadow of death, and souls
departed but the shadows of the living.'
– Thomas Brown

It was a very busy Wednesday morning on 14 December 2011 in the Clinical & Forensic Medicine Unit (CFMU) at the Sydney Police Centre, Surry Hills, and I had a large number of DUIDs (driving under the influence of drugs) to attend to. The 'In' tray was overflowing and I was beginning to become a bit stressed from the amount of work I had to deal with and wondering which ones to prioritise … when the telephone rang.

'Could you check this one out doc?' was the police initial enquiry.

After talking to the detective involved in the case for some time on the telephone, I soon realised there was little evidence to work on for this matter.

I protested, 'But there's only skeletal remains. I'm a toxicologist and there's only bones to test.' Eventually, I relented and said, 'Well, is there any hair available to be tested?'

He was affirmative and agreed to have the hair from the deceased tested for drugs.

The case was now in my hands from a forensic toxicological perspective. I took his details, and mailed a test kit to him which contained instructions on how to sample the hair from the remains for testing at the laboratory.

Mr Andrew Drake was a homeless person who lived in a cave near the Three Sisters rock formation at Echo Point, Katoomba, New South Wales. On 10 December 2011, it was an unusually cool summer morning for the time of the year with the temperature hovering around 18 degrees Celsius, when he was foraging around the bushland looking for old bottles to supplement his meagre income. Shortly before midday, he made his way up the side of a very steep bush section below the Echo Point Lookout. As he stopped to gather his breath, he noticed something lying in the undergrowth. As he drew near, he saw that it was an intact human skeleton. Due to the extent of decomposition, the body had clearly been there for some time. After taking a few minutes to recover from his shock, Mr Drake went to the Katoomba Police Station and reported his grisly find.

Officers of the Police Rescue Squad were mobilised and able to recover the skeletal remains the next day. These were packaged and appropriately labelled and conveyed to the Glebe Mortuary. On 14 December 2011 the skeletal remains were subsequently identified as being those of Mrs Margaret Elizabeth Hills through examination of dental records by Dr Alain Middleton, a senior forensic odontologist and reports from Dr Isabella Brouwer, forensic pathologist and Dr Denise Donlon, forensic anthropologist who confirmed the presence of surgical pins and plates in her vertebral column. Mrs Hills' medical records showed that some years earlier following work injuries, she had undergone spinal surgery that involved the insertion of surgical pins and plates.

Margaret Elizabeth Hills was born on 18 July 1949 and her disappearance had been previously reported by her husband Kenneth

Hills on 2 February 2010. Mr Hills told police that she had been home when he had gone to bed, but was not at their Katoomba home when he awoke. He said that he had tried to find her in the usual places but was unsuccessful. Further, extensive searches for her were carried out by both the police and other public authorities along with members of Mrs Hills' family. Curiously, she had left home without her medication nor any money.

Prior to her death, Mrs Hills was employed as a receptionist at the World Square development site in George Street, Sydney. On 10 November 2000 she was collecting mail from the security office on the ground floor of the building. As she was returning to her office, a reversing truck dislodged a piece of concrete structure which hit a rail that knocked her off her feet. She landed heavily onto the concrete floor injuring her left hip and buttock. In addition, she suffered from a severe back injury which needed repeated surgery and the insertion of screws and plates. As a consequence, she experienced constant pain, difficulties with her balance necessitating the use of a walking stick and suffered from depression. It was a very difficult time for Margaret Hills.

Strike Force Tapley was formed to investigate Mrs Margaret Hills' disappearance which was so out of character for her. Something was clearly amiss. However, she was not found until, Mr Drake's gruesome discovery on that cool December morning in 2011.

Katoomba is the main town in the Blue Mountains of New South Wales. The town name is derived from the Aboriginal term Kedumba or Katta-toon-bah meaning 'shining, falling water' or 'water tumbling over hill' and is derived from the waterfall that drops into the Jamison Valley below the Harrys Amphitheatre escarpment. It is the administrative headquarters of the Blue Mountains City Council.

The spot where Mr Drake found Mrs Hills' remains at Echo Point lookout is about 2 kilometres south of Katoomba. It is a popular tourist attraction with up to two million visitors each year. The lookout provides an excellent view of the Three Sisters, three ancient weathered sandstone peaks formed many thousands of years ago through erosion, along with other rock formations such as the Ruined Castle and Mount Solitary.

An analysis of the hair sample (taken because no suitable body tissues and/or fluids were available) proved to be inconclusive. This was most likely due several factors including the lengthy time interval and exposure to weathering, possibly resulting in leaching of any substances of interest.

In the meantime, the police investigation continued after Mrs Hills' remains were discovered. Then, at 6.15 am on Saturday 1 September 2012, following a two-and-a-half year investigation, detectives arrested Ken Hills at his Ingleburn home in Sydney's south-west, which he shared with his de facto. He was taken to Macquarie Fields Police Station and charged with his wife's murder and bailed to appear in Parramatta Court the following day. It is the right of every person in New South Wales who has been charged and refused bail by police to face court within 24 hours. It is a requirement that the accused person has had the opportunity to apply for bail before a magistrate.

On 28 September 2012 an inquest before Mr Paul MacMahon, Deputy State Coroner was commenced at the Coroner's Court in Glebe. Mr MacMahon was subsequently advised by the Director of Public Prosecutions that they had decided to discontinue the indictable proceedings that had been commenced against Kenneth Hills, as there appeared to be insufficient evidence available. And so, the inquest was resumed before Mr MacMahon at Katoomba on 3 November 2014. The inquest continued until 14 November 2014. A voluminous brief of evidence was assembled by the police and various other witnesses involved in the investigation.

The coroner found that there were a number of factors which indicated the possibility that Mrs Hills' death was self-inflicted given she was suffering from depression. This seemed to be supported by one witness, Mr Robert Deahm, a fellow parishioner of Mrs Hills, at the Anglican Church at Wentworth Falls, where he saw her at a Sunday service just before she disappeared. She appeared very unhappy and during their conversation she said a number of times, 'I just wish the Lord would take me.'

Further, another witness, Melissa Taylor described on 30 January 2010 when she was driving along Megalong Street, Leura, Mrs Hills stepped straight onto the road in front of her. She had to brake hard so that she did not hit her. Ms Taylor said that Mrs Hills had a 'vacant' look about her, like someone with major depression or dementia.

However, these did not explain how a woman in pain, shuffling along with a walking stick could get to Echo Point, some 3 kilometres from her home, where the terrain at times is quite steep. Further, even if she was able to get to Echo Point unaided, it didn't explain how her body got to the location where it was found.

If she had jumped from the lower viewing platform above where her remains were found below, it appeared difficult to discern how her body reached its final resting place because of the presence of a ledge between the possible jumping places and where her body lay. Also, assuming she had jumped from the lower viewing platform, it would be expected for her body to have significant fractures or other physical damage. There was none.

Unable to determine either the manner or cause of Margaret Hills' death, the deputy coroner returned an open verdict, meaning the case remained open, however Kenneth Hills was 'identified as being a person of sufficient interest'. He was granted leave to appear at the inquest and was represented by Counsel throughout the proceedings.

So if you the reader have any information that may help investigators to close this cold case and bring the perpetrator(s) to justice, please call Crime Stoppers on 1800 333 000.

26 Magic Mushrooms

'It is funny how those substances
[from 'magic mushrooms'] could distort your mind,
from the clear and straight one, into something else
you never imagined before.'
– Rima Reyka

A number of hallucinogens are known to occur in nature, including dimethyltryptamine (DMT) from salvia (*Salvia divinorum*, a herbal mint plant from the sage family and many other plants), mescaline (from the peyote cactus), lysergic acid (a precursor to LSD) produced by the ergot fungus that often grows on the cereal, rye – and in this case, psilocybin, or 'magic mushrooms'. Psilocybin or psilocin are hallucinogenic substances found in over one hundred species of mushrooms worldwide. These mushrooms are found in the wild and are also cultivated. The cultivated mushrooms tend to be more potent through selection of stronger mushroom strains (a similar approach is used in cannabis cultivation).

The more well-known species are the gold top mushrooms (*Psilocybe cubensis*) and Mexican mushrooms (*Psilocybe mexicana*). The latter were used by Mexican Indians in their various shaman religious ceremonies. However, it is the former that is the most well-known due to its wide distribution and ease of cultivation. The mushroom (or toadstool) quite often resembles the common field mushroom (*Psalliota campestris*) in general appearance but generally grows in clumps on cow dung. The stalks are quite thin, with a ring of tissue (veil) just below the cap. The cap is whitish when young which becomes a golden light-tan colour when mature, giving rise to the more common names 'golden tops', 'gold caps' and due to their hallucinogenic effects, 'magic mushrooms' and 'shrooms'. Quite often, because the fungi are found growing in the wild, magic mushrooms are considered a safe alternative to harder drugs such as MDMA (ecstasy). However, there are still risks associated with consuming these psychedelic fungi. Along with varying dosages of the hallucinogenic component, there is always the problem of a 'bad trip' (very much like that experienced by users of LSD). This may involve unpleasant physical symptoms such as chills, nausea and vomiting. Other unwanted side-effects may include negative psychological effects such as paranoia and severe anxiety leading to panic attacks. Generally, users of magic mushrooms welcome the hallucinations and the sense of altered reality that ingestion of the fungi can bring about. But, this altered perception of their surroundings can potentially cause the users to take unusual risks and/or unknowingly place themselves into dangerous situations.

Not a good place to be, whatever activity you plan to do.

★

It was another busy Monday morning on 11 April 2011 when I received a curious request from a police officer about an exhibit of magic mushrooms. It appeared a young couple were apprehended by police and were found in possession of two quantities of fresh mushrooms (46 grams and 345 grams respectively) weighing a total of 391 grams, just over a year earlier (14 October 2010).

Mushrooms, mushrooms – so what was the big deal? But this mushroom cache was quite different. It was no grocery item!

They were fresh 'gold top' mushrooms. The hallucinogenic kind and were identified as the *Psilocybe cubensis* species. The fungi were subsequently analysed and, sure enough, found to contain psilocin.

I subsequently reported that psilocin is the dephosphorylated analogue of psilocybin which is a naturally occurring tryptamine derivative that has been used as a drug of abuse. It is typically encountered as the fresh or dried *Psilocybe cubensis* mushroom, which may be directly ingested orally or brewed as a tea. Due to its bitter taste it is sometimes incorporated into a chocolate mix to make it easier to consume.

A 1 gram portion of the fungi material typically provides about 10 milligrams of psilocybin, and when ingested, the phosphate group is metabolically removed (in the liver) producing the active drug, psilocin.

I then explained that, psilocin is a psychoactive drug that causes perceptual distortion, confusion, agitation, hallucinations, hyperactivity, hysterical behaviour and delirium. The greatest danger associated with consumption of the drug is the antisocial behaviour that can occur, and similar to LSD, a phenomena known a 'flashbacks' may persist some months after usage.

Further questions were raised by the Department of Public Prosecutions (DPP) no doubt, in an effort to determine how to run their case before court.

I was asked, 'How long after consumption of the mushrooms do the psychoactive effects begin?'

And I answered, 'This depends upon how the fungi are consumed. Psilocybin is absorbed through the lining of the mouth and stomach. If the user chews on the fungi or holds them in their mouth for a few minutes, the effects of the drug begin in about 10 minutes. However, eating and swallowing the fungi delay the effects for about 30–40 minutes. When the psilocybin passes through the digestive system and into the liver, it is metabolised [changed] into psilocin, the pharmacologically active drug form.'

I was then asked how long the effects last and said, 'The effects last from two to six hours depending upon dosage.'

This was followed up by, 'How much of the active drug needs to be consumed in order to induce psychoactive effects?'

I replied, 'A typical single, oral hallucinogenic recreational dose of psilocybin is 10 milligrams, which may be found in a gram of fresh *Psilocybe cubensis* fungi. However, this can range from 10 to 50 milligrams psilocybin [equivalent to 1 to 5 grams of fresh fungi], although only 4 to 10 milligrams are required for the hallucinogenic effects.'

The next questions were to determine if personal use of the quantity was reasonable. Could one person be expected to consume the 345-gram bag of mushrooms within a 72-hour period? (There was a weight difference of 46 grams, which I assumed was probably due to loss of moisture while in storage. In any case it worked in the defendant's favour.)

I answered, 'A recreational dose of psilocybin is usually 10 milligrams and can range up to 50 milligrams of the drug. This would be about equivalent to 1 to 5 grams of fresh fungi. Therefore, if 345 grams of fungi are allegedly consumed over 72 hours – three days – this would be equivalent to the consumption of 115 grams of fresh fungi – magic mushrooms – per day or 23 times the top of recreational usage.'

Clearly, this regimen was unlikely. However, the DPP persisted in this line of questioning,

'If a person did consume the 345-gram bag of mushrooms within a 72-hour period, what would he expect to be the likely effects of the drug upon that person?

I paused for a moment and reflected on the question, 'Well, assuming the fungi were fresh, this alleged consumption is excessive. The adverse effects from excessive consumption of psilocybin include anxiety, paranoid delusions, depersonalisation, dilated pupils, disorientation, hallucinations, vomiting, tachycardia and paraesthesia.' (Abnormal sensations for example, prickling, sensation of insects such ants on the skin etc.)

I concluded the mushrooms did not appear to be just for personal use.

The magic mushrooms came under the *Drug Misuse and Trafficking Act 1985* Schedule 1 which describes 'Prohibited plant or prohibited drug' where 'Psilocin and its derivatives being those derivatives having hallucinogenic properties'.

Under the Act, an amount of this drug being 100 grams or more, was considered a 'large commercial quantity' namely, 'The quantity specified above (if any) of the drug to which the analogous substance is related (or, if there is more than one such drug, the largest among the quantities specified above (if any) of those drugs).'

This information appeared to be enough for the DPP and my statement was tendered to the court. Surprisingly, I wasn't called to give evidence for this matter. Maybe they thought the contents of the statement were sufficient to proceed.

In any case, with the possession of 345 grams of the magic mushrooms, over three times the 'large commercial quantity', the couple were clearly in trouble with the law. In New South Wales the possession of a drug (for your own personal use) is a summary offence, which means it is handled at local court level. This carries a maximum penalty of $2200 and/or imprisonment for two years.

Because they were found with a larger amount of drug, they were 'deemed to possess the drugs for the purpose of supplying them' which meant they would have automatically faced much higher penalties, unless they were able to prove that the drugs were for their own use, which would have been difficult.

My evidence may have been quite damaging.

I later spoke to the Department of Public Prosecutions and asked what sentence would be appropriate for an offence of that nature and they indicated at least a period of penal servitude.

The couple were very lucky, instead they received a hefty fine but, no jail time.

The 'Ice Man' Cometh: The Jessica Silva Case

'Meth takes you down one of three roads:
jail, the psych ward, or death.'
– Lauren Myacle

Twenty-two-year-old Jessica Silva and her de facto husband, James Polkinghorne, six years her senior, had a very volatile relationship; it was a real love/hate affair. Their time together, which produced a child, oscillated between bouts of torrid love making and angry slanging matches – 'fire and ice' served up on a bed of smouldering emotion.

But that was nothing compared to the more deadly form of ice that entered their lives. That ice was not of the frozen watery kind, but the nasty dangerous drug, methylamphetamine, which resembles ice in its purest and most potent form.

Jessica told her friends that she'd been verbally and physically abused and that she feared for her life, as James was not only selling the drug, but also consuming it.

It was a recipe for disaster and further damaged their already shaky four-year alliance. Eventually, the years of extreme domestic abuse made

Jessica decide that enough was enough and she moved out of the family home and in with her parents until she could find her feet and alternative accommodation.

Unfortunately, that was not the end of the matter. Unknown to Jessica at the time, James had become a prime police suspect in a drug murder, and he started calling her, making taunts, such as 'Jessica, do you know who I am? I'm a fucking murderer,' something which was to become vital evidence in future court proceedings.

High on ice and increasingly paranoid and aggressive, James called her again. It was 11 May 2012, two days before Mother's Day. On that occasion, he made a threat, saying, 'I'll kill youse all. I'm telling you, I'm not fucking joking.'

Matters came to a head on Mother's Day, when at about 9 pm, James called in at Jessica's parents' address in Marrickville, turning what was supposed to be the conclusion to a friendly family celebration into something that was quite the opposite. Once again, he was high on ice, and before arriving at the house, he'd given Jessica a taste of what to expect by texting, 'I hope your mother gets poisoned by the flowers that you give her and you get gang raped. If you are alive (tomorrow) I'm caving your face.'

Unsurprisingly, on his arrival, an altercation broke out between him and a couple of Silva family members, namely Jessica's brother, Miguel, and her father, Avalino, who tried to restrain him. He allegedly attacked Jessica, ripping her pants, and she ran inside the family home, where she retrieved a large kitchen knife with which to defend herself and her family members. When she returned to the scene, she grappled with James and allegedly stabbed him four or five times to the back and shoulder areas.

In spite of his wounds, while struggling to get up from the road, he screamed, 'Kill! I'm gonna kill youse.' He then collapsed and died where he lay, and after the authorities had been notified and gone through the usual procedures, his body was taken to the Royal Prince Alfred Hospital. Jessica was arrested by police and later charged with his murder.

A blood sample taken from James at the post-mortem was found to have present methylamphetamine (ice) 0.21 milligrams per litre and amphetamine 0.09 milligrams per litre. The latter drug is also a metabolite of methylamphetamine and indicated that the drug had been in his body for some time. But more importantly, the level of methylamphetamine present in his blood was well above the therapeutic or feel-good level sought by users of the drug. He'd clearly developed a tolerance to the drug, but not to its aggressive qualities. The post-mortem injuries showed the actual cause of his death was through stabbing injuries and not from an overdose of methylamphetamine.

Jessica spent 29 weeks in the maximum-security Silverwater prison before her trial on 12 November 2014, although by the time the trial by jury in the Supreme Court began, she'd been released from prison and was out on bail.

The issue at hand was did she commit murder, manslaughter or was it self-defence?

She pleaded not guilty to the charges of murder and manslaughter.

On 2 December, the jury heard evidence regarding the savage, cruel and degrading domestic abuse that she'd been subjected to for years. Then on 4 December, after the prosecution had said that there were lawful ways to respond to domestic violence, the jury found her not guilty of murder but guilty of manslaughter. On hearing the verdict, Jessica collapsed in the dock. She was subsequently sentenced to 18 months in jail, although the sentence was wholly suspended by Supreme Court Justice Clifton Hoeben, who found

'... the death was committed under extreme circumstances in the agony of the moment.'

However, Jessica was keen to clear her name, and on 27 June 2016, she appealed to the Court of Criminal Appeal to have the manslaughter conviction overturned and her name cleared, arguing that she'd been acting in self-defence.

On 7 December, the Court of Criminal Appeal surprisingly overturned her conviction, although it was a non-unanimous decision. Justice Lucy McCallum stated that, 'Ms Silva can only have perceived the deceased's attack on her that evening as urgent, life-threatening and inescapable.'

Subsequently, the court ordered a judgment and a verdict of acquittal to be entered.

Jessica's lawyer, Adam Houda, declared that his client had been 'emphatically cleared of any wrongdoing'.

One positive arising from the case was that it raised the profile of the issue of domestic violence.

Jessica had been forced to leave James Polkinghorne because he'd been abusive and had threatened to kill her. And worse still, he'd found the safe place she'd run to. However, although she acted in self-defence, as the Crown pointed out, there were other avenues open to deal with such domestic violence, and an apprehended violence order (AVO) and police intervention may well have prevented the bloodshed that resulted.

I personally feel the latter approach would have been more helpful. AVOs tend to inflame an already volatile situation.

The Barbieri Bastion: A Fortress of Fear

'There can be heroism in the moment,
but courage is always in the day-to-day.'
– Robert Brault

Oakville is a delightful outer western suburb of Sydney. It has the best of both worlds with a country town atmosphere, but also the advantages of proximity to the city. It is located about 50 kilometres north-west of the Sydney central business district and in the local government area of the City of Hawkesbury. In the 2016 census, the urban centre of Oakville was recorded as having a population of 1964. For most visitors, it is an opportunity to relax and enjoy the Hawkesbury Valley's peaceful farming community where large roadside fruit and vegetable shops display excellent produce from the farms. A true treat, certainly for families from the city wishing to purchase fresh produce from the farm gate at very reasonable prices.

And if that isn't enough, the hospital (Clare House) in Oakville is well known for its use as the Wandin Valley Bush Nursing Hospital' in the long-running Channel 7 television series *A Country Practice,* which ran for 12 years (1981–1993). In addition, Oakville had a family score of 8/10 as a place to live and a tranquillity score of 9/10. But more importantly, it had a safety score of 10/10. Apparently, a wonderful safe place to live.

So, it was in this most unlikely country setting that this story of madness, murder and heroism was to unfold.

★

As in many communities there are families that have a number of serious problems. Sometimes self-inflicted, some genetic, poor planning or just down right unlucky.

The Barbieri family had a number of problems, which appeared to be mental-health issues that spilled out onto their neighbour, the Waters family, with disastrous results.

But this wasn't always so.

Born in February 1967, Fiona Barbieri (nee Champley) eventually made a successful career working for American Express, after trying her hand at secretarial work. The company appreciated her efforts so much that in 1998 they promoted her to program manager and transferred her, her husband Angelo Barbieri and their son, Mitchell, then five years old, to an Amex headquarters in Phoenix, Arizona. Unfortunately, the Barbieri family only stayed in the United States for a few months, returning to Australia when Fiona learned that one of her sisters was diagnosed with leukaemia. Then towards the end of 2000, the Barbieris purchased a 5-acre property at 33 Scheyville Road, Oakville. Fiona Barbieri still had her job with Amex, but worked through the night from home so that she could stay on American time. It was a difficult, but workable arrangement.

In the meantime, in 2002, tow-truck king Kevin Waters purchased a property next to the Barbieris and initially the two neighbours got along well. In addition, Waters being a bird fancier, now had enough room for several aviaries which housed a variety of exotic birds and hundreds of pigeons.

Then, in 2003, Fiona and Angelo divorced. She kept the house having taking over the mortgage. Fiona Barbieri later took in a boyfriend and the couple got engaged. This occurred while Mitchell (sometimes called Mitch) was at Bede Polding College at Bligh Park, a Catholic co-educational secondary school, located at South Windsor about a 14-minute drive from Oakville. The school's motto is 'Called to Bring Peace', a motto that was to prove somewhat ironic for Mitchell, after his mother's fiancée bought him a compound bow!

A compound bow is a bow that uses a levering system, usually of cables and pulleys, to bend the limbs. Generally, compound bows are used in target practice and hunting. Due to this technology, an archer is able to point an arrow at a target and with some training, actually hit the target with a high degree of accuracy. Mitchell practised with the weapon and soon became quite proficient.

In 2008, the romance between Fiona and her boyfriend over, the fiancé moved out and the hosting of wild parties moved in. Here, Fiona Barbieri began her rants to her young guests about government conspiracies and neighbours through a 'mental mist' of alcohol and a cloud of cannabis smoke. Mitch was subsequently expelled from school after an indiscreet posting of slanderous videos on YouTube about the school principal. He subsequently moved on to Hawkesbury High School. In the meantime, Fiona and Mitch began turning their house into a fortress, collecting an arsenal of barbaric weapons which included a selection of samurai swords, a barbed wire garrotte, a rope flail, baseball bats and an assortment of hunting knives. In addition, outside the house, they had placed a number of concealed mantraps, wooden boards with 10 cm nails sticking out designed to maim any intruder on the property. Mother and son rarely left the house or went anywhere without each other, and withdrew from the outside world which they saw full of enemies – including the police.

In 2009, Fiona Barbieri's mental health was rapidly deteriorating, where she was becoming more paranoid and took an overdose of prescription tablets in a suicide attempt. It was Mr Waters who arrived in time, called the paramedics, and saved her life. Even so, she still regarded him as an enemy. As the year rolled on, friends noticed that Fiona was neglecting her hygiene and appearance and towards the end of 2009 she went on permanent sick leave from American Express. She was later made redundant and left Amex with a substantial pay out. The following year,

Fiona Barbieri was diagnosed with bipolar disorder and told her doctor that Kevin Waters was harassing them because he wanted them to leave and then purchase their property at well below market value. However, her perceived problems not only included her neighbour, but her former employer, Amex and various 'government and non-government conspiracies'.

By 2011, the Barbieris spent most of their days smoking cannabis and had become more paranoid and reclusive, even neglecting family and friends. Excessive cannabis use is known to exacerbate underlying psychotic conditions. By now, Fiona Barbieri's redundancy payment was spent and being ineligible for Centrelink payments, the bills began to mount up. The first to go was the electricity supply and this was not reconnected. However, to maintain their water supply, the water meter was wrapped in barbed wire to prevent a reading.

The house and gardens had become neglected and Barbieris were now living in virtual squalor, depending upon candles at night for light and the generosity of friends for the occasional hot shower. To further add to their woes, the Commonwealth Bank began actions to foreclose on the mortgage on their property.

Still they continued to smoke cannabis and their relationship with Kevin Waters further deteriorated, peaking on the evening of 3 December 2012. Mr Waters was in his house when he heard a loud thud outside the window. He looked out and saw a light from the Barbieri property and heard Mitchell Barbieri call out, 'We will rebuke you.' The following morning Kevin Waters found a stick with a note attached saying the words Mitchell had said the previous evening. However, it was not the first time that sticks had been thrown onto his property by the 'nutter' Barbieris.

In the meantime, mother and son put up signs around their property warning: 'We will rebuke you', then placed a sign on the closed and locked gate that read: 'Autarchy in place on these premises, strictly appointment only'. Autarchy meant that they were asserting absolute sovereignty or self-government on the property.

With backup weapons, which included several sledge hammers, a gas bottle kitted out as a flame thrower, swords, knives and two savage

Neapolitan mastiff dogs ready for duty.

The Barbieri bastion, now a fortress of fear, was complete.

Not surprisingly, Mr Waters was becoming increasingly concerned about the safety of his family and himself. He decided to employ an electrician to install flood lights around his property to alert him of any night time intruders. It was about midday on 6 December 2012 when electrician Peter Yard began installing floodlights near a number of aviaries that were located several metres away from the Barbieris' boundary. Shortly after he began work Fiona Barbieri came to the fence line and started abusing Mr Yard, who then returned to the house to let Mr Waters know what was going on. Later, he returned with a fellow worker, Kevin West, to complete the job. Unfortunately, Fiona Barbieri was now armed with a baseball bat, demanded that the ladder and equipment be removed. But more chillingly, Mitchell Barbieri had now joined the fray and aimed his compound bow and arrow at Mr Yard and Mr West, who, seeing the danger, quickly sought cover just as an arrow was released from the bow. The arrow narrowly missed the men close to chest height, and struck a nearby wall.

On hearing the ruckus, Mr Waters and his son emerged from the house to assist Mr Yard and Mr West, followed by another employee, Damien Roe, who decided to record the subsequent events on his mobile phone. Again, on seeing further targets, Michell Barbieri aimed his bow and arrow at Kevin and Kurt Waters. Fortunately, the arrow narrowly missed the men, this time landing in the ground close by where they were standing. A further arrow was released before the men bolted to safety.

But enough, was enough.

The men had retreated into the house and triple-O was called, with the police being requested to attend the Oakville address.

The stage was now set for a tragic showdown.

The incident was recorded on police radio just after 2 pm 'as a person shooting arrows from a bow at a neighbour'. A police car acknowledged the call and proceeded to the Waters' property. On arrival, Constables James Ghata and Hannah Watson proceeded to take statements from the witnesses, while seeing the arrows in the backyard.

In the meantime, the Barbieris had retreated inside their barricaded home and began sending numerous emails to federal and state ministers titled: 'BARBIERI versus WATERS' claiming they were being provoked and intimidated. One email said, 'Let me remind you, we have every right to defend ourselves, our family and our property.'

At just after quarter past two that afternoon, Detective Senior Constables Caulfield and Ornatowski arrived with Senior Constable Jonathon Hughes. Constable Ghata gave them an update on what was happening at the property.

The detectives walked up to the locked front gate of the Barbieris and tried to gain their attention. Mitchell Barbieri was briefly seen at the window of the house with a camera and was asked to come out. There was no response.

The police officers realised that it was too dangerous to attempt entry into the premises without backup. In addition, Detective Ornatowski requested a search warrant application to allow police to search for the offending bow and arrow – and no doubt, other weapons.

At 2.55 pm the Barbieris sent another email which said, 'Our property is surrounded', adding, 'Corrupt police attempting to break in to our property whilst Waters front yard is full of drivers and associates. We have photographic evidence. Tell them to put in writing we know how the corrupt system works now.' A few minutes later, Detective Ornatowski requested further backup to the area.

At 3.11 pm another email was sent by the Barbieris to the same politicians, as three more police cars arrived: 'What reinforcements arriving???' Further adding, 'What sending reinforcements to target/ ambush the innocent mother and son that our Government offered up to be murdered? Do you know you don't sacrifice the innocent?'

At 3.12 pm, just only a minute later, Mitchell Barbieri texted his father saying: 'The Police are at the front gate. For standing up for our rights.' His father replied, 'Don't do anything silly, see what they want.'

Sadly, that very wise piece of advice did not reach his son.

It appeared a siege situation had now set in – and it was not a good look.

Sergeant Fitzgibbon then decided to return to Windsor Police Station to get tasers, as none of the police there had one. Before departing he instructed the officers to maintain a safe distance from the Barbieri premises, and to hold their positions making sure that no-one entered nor anyone left the premises. With that, Sergeant Fitzgibbon left with Detective Caulfield to collect the necessary equipment from the police station. During the trip back to the station Windsor police were briefed about the ' … possible siege situation and the occupants were refusing to speak to police' prior to being told the Oakville address.

Back at Windsor Police Station, Detective Inspector Bryson Anderson told Detective Caulfield and Inspector Battin that he had a number of dealings with Barbieris, recognising they had mental health issues. And noted there were about 38 COPS (Computer Operated Policing System) events recorded against the Barbieris, all relating to events that occurred on their Oakville property. Most of these were relatively minor events such as improper use of emails, an assault and so on. But these were seen to escalate to incidents involving domestic violence, malicious damage and the ever-present complaints against neighbours. Apparently, one report recorded that Mitchell Barbieri could be suicidal and had access to hunting knives.

Curiously, there were no warnings referring to Mitchell Barbieri's mental problems nor the presence of the two aggressive large dogs.

Still strenuous efforts were taken to resolve the situation in a peaceful manner.

At about quarter to four, Detective Ornatowski who was at the front gate of the Barbieri property, used a loud speaker attached to a police vehicle to address the Barbieris saying, 'Mitchell, Fiona, it's the police. You aren't in trouble; we just need to talk to you about what happened today.'

There was no response, apart from the dogs barking loudly.

Apparently, Detective Inspector Anderson was heard to say, 'Well we are getting no response from out here so we will try to knock on the door.'

At close to 4 pm, there was a suggestion to get the Tactical Operations Unit and negotiators in to deal with the situation. After much to and froing, nothing much seemed to be achieved. Then at 4.08 pm Detective

Inspector Anderson sent a text message to Inspector Battin saying, 'One very big dog inside and they're [the Barbieris] staying staunch.'

Unfortunately, there was again no response.

At about 4.14 pm Inspector Bryson Anderson along with four police officers at the back of the Barbieri house, made the fateful decision to go in saying.

In the meantime, Inspector Battin was on the mobile phone expressing his concerns about the police going in without backup. Sergeant McCormack replied, 'Are you sure about that?' Inspector Battin then says, 'We've got vested-up police to go in and physically engage him. I am happy with it because one of these guys [Anderson] knows this guy.'

This could not have been further from the truth. They were in fact, dealing with people with serious mental issues, and as such totally unpredictable.

Nevertheless, Sergeant Fitzgibbon kicked the rear door open.

As the door was flung open, two massive, aggressive dogs rushed out onto the verandah barking and generally carrying on. They were in turn, greeted with a hefty dose of capsicum spray onto the animals delivered by police officers, Ghata, Camilleri, and Watson, followed later by Ornatowski. However, in the confined space a number of officers were also incapacitated.

Unfortunately, Mitchell Barbieri had also followed the dogs, armed with a 27-cm hunting knife. In a lunging motion, he stabbed Inspector Bryson Anderson in the top right of his chest and then into his face, while his mother swung a 1.8-kg block hammer at other police officers who attempted to intervene.

The deep wound to Inspector Anderson's chest was to prove fatal.

Almost immediately, Mitchell Barbieri was flung to the ground by accompanying police officers. In the process, the blood stained knife was knocked from his hand. Even so, it took some time to subdue him and his mother, while they shouted out their verbal barrage of abuse. They were subsequently arrested, handcuffed and taken out to the police vehicles.

At 4.16 pm, police called for urgent assistance and an ambulance, as an officer had been struck down and required urgent medical attention. In the meantime, fellow officers rushed to Inspector Anderson's aid. They were able to speak to him briefly, before he lapsed into unconsciousness.

At 4.25 pm, ambulance officers arrived at the scene and worked on the stricken police officer in an attempt to stabilise him before being transferred to Hawkesbury Hospital. Then at 5.03 pm, despite the best efforts of the medical team, Detective Inspector Anderson tragically passed away.

On the morning of 7 December 2012 Dr Istvan Szentmariay, forensic pathologist, performed a post-mortem on Detective Inspector Anderson at the Department of Forensic Medicine, Glebe. He found that the police officer had died as a result of a 14 cm stab wound to the chest.

A Critical Incident Investigation Team in accordance with NSWPF guidelines, was formed to investigate the death of Detective Inspector Bryson Charles Anderson, as he was killed in the line of duty.

Blood samples were taken from all parties concerned including, the deceased.

Only a therapeutic level of the drug venlafaxine (commonly known as Efexor) was detected in Inspector Anderson's blood sample. The drug is used to treat anxiety and depression. Given his stressful position, I believed this was an appropriate medication.

Not surprisingly, cannabis residues were detected in both Mitchell and Fiona Barbieri's blood samples, given their previous history. However, I was of the opinion that the cannabinoids detected in the Barbieris' blood samples were too low to impact on their behaviour at the time of the incident.

Detective Inspector Bryson Anderson's death touched everyone particularly, those who worked with him at Windsor Police Station, and his fellow officers wanted to honour their fallen comrade in a special way.

On a warm, sunny afternoon of Wednesday 12 December 2012, family and friends of Detective Anderson gathered to mourn and farewell the fallen officer at Parramatta, in western Sydney. The procession to the church included police cars (one marked with the number plate 'BCA 12'), motorbikes and numerous police on foot. A full police funeral took place, including marching escorts, hundreds of police colleagues and a roadside guard of honour, which formed outside St Patrick's Cathedral.

At the conclusion of the service, the funeral procession with a marching escort travelled along Victoria Road between Marist Place and O'Connell Street.

It was a huge turnout and a 'sea of blue' from all the uniformed police officers who attended.

Police aircraft (PolAir helicopters) also joined in a salute from the air, and the NSW Governor, Dame Marie Bashir, along with many politicians, including NSW Premier, Mr Barry O'Farrell, attended, along with representatives from the NSW ambulance services and NSW fire brigades.

The NSW Police Commissioner, Mr Andrew Scipione, had the unenviable task to read a second valedictory for another fallen police officer in the same year, alongside a eulogy for the Anderson family. Detective Inspector Bryson Charles Anderson was awarded two posthumous medals, the National Police Service Medal: 'recognising Bryson's ethical and diligent service in protecting the community.' And the Commissioner's Valour Award (VA): 'For conspicuous action and exceptional courage he displayed at the incident in Oakville where he lost his life. After being attacked with a knife and sustaining wounds that would prove fatal, Detective Inspector Anderson went to the aid of a fellow injured officer without hesitation.'

In part the valour citation read: 'Conferred for conspicuous merit and exceptional bravery whilst under attack during the execution of his duties at Oakville on Thursday, 6 December 2012.'

It was a deeply moving speech describing a talented, dedicated police officer. A devoted husband and father – and also his dedication to community service. Adding, 'A thoroughly good bloke.'

Because a police officer had been killed, the matter became a very high profile case.

It was to be two years later on Wednesday 5 November 2014, when the matter went before the Supreme Court in Sydney for sentencing before Justice Robert Hulme. Previously, both mother and son had been charged with murder over the killing. In a courtroom packed with the police officer's family, friends and his former police colleagues, Mitchell Barbieri and his mother, Fiona Barbieri, pleaded guilty to their crimes.

Mitchell Barbieri faced a mandatory life sentence in jail (as was the case in the Senior Constable David Rixon murder earlier) where a police officer is murdered in the course of his or her duty. However, the court heard before Justice Hulme and the Crown accepted the plea of manslaughter for Fiona Barbieri on the grounds that she was suffering 'a substantial impairment brought about by an abnormality of mind'. She was said have had paranoid schizophrenia at the time of the offence and was sentenced to a minimum of seven years and six months for the manslaughter of the police officer and a number of other offences.

The following day, Justice Hulme found that Mitchell Barbieri had intended to kill Inspector Anderson on the day of the incident commenting, 'Of all the weapons that he could have taken up, he chose the one most capable of inflicting a lethal injury.' He considered Mitchell's cognitive impairment and decided that he should not be subject to a mandatory life sentence for a person found guilty of murdering an on-duty police officer. Instead, he sentenced him to a minimum of 26 years and a maximum of 35 years, making him eligible for release in 2038. He broke down when the sentence was handed down.

Outside court a very disappointed Mrs Donna Anderson said, 'We will still wake tomorrow without Bryson.' Adding, 'Not one of us has been left unchanged by this senseless act,' and acknowledging that no sentence would have been sufficient for the crime committed.

Unfortunately, for the Anderson family, this was not the end of the legal process.

On Monday 12 December 2016 the matter went before the NSW Court of Criminal Appeal where Mitchell Barbieri appealed against his sentence citing that his mental health issues had not been adequately considered.

The court heard that Fiona Barbieri was suffering from paranoid schizophrenia at the time and her son had 'a transferred delusional disorder' from her. In the judgment Justice Carolyn Simpson found the sentencing judge had erred when considering Mitchell Barbieri's 'plainly severe' mental illness. She added, that it made no difference that his mental illness was 'secondary' or a 'derivative' from his mother. Further adding, 'His mental illness diminished his moral culpability to a very significant degree.'

The final outcome was that Mitchell Barbieri had 11 years cut from his non-parole period. He was re-sentenced to at least 15 years jail, with a maximum term of 21 years and three months.

Justice Derek Price was the dissenting judge and said Barbieri should be re-sentenced to a maximum of 32 years. However, the previous ruling was handed down.

It was another disappointment for the Anderson family.

Inspector Anderson's brother, Warwick, commented outside court that the decision was, '… beyond belief'. Saying, 'We came here today and were − to use my father's words − kicked in the guts by the decision handed down today.'

The NSW Police Commissioner Andrew Scipione wrote to the Director of Public Prosecutions, Mr Lloyd Babb, SC to initiate an appeal in the High Court. He also commented, 'The police family are hurting, none more so than the family of Bryson.'

Mr Babb in turn, took the matter to the High Court arguing that the decision '… failed to properly apply the principle of deterrence'. But the High Court subsequently refused to hear the appeal against sentence reduction for Mitchell Barbieri killing Detective Inspector Bryson Anderson.

And there the matter stood.

It was now necessary to work out what went terribly wrong and how to ensure it didn't happen again. To achieve this, an inquest into the murder of Detective Inspector Bryson Anderson was held on 19 June 2018 at Glebe Coroner's Court before the Deputy State Coroner O'Sullivan. Some six years after his murder.

Before a packed court, the counsel assisting the coroner, Dr Peggy Dwyer, praised Inspector Anderson who had courageously put himself on the frontline during the siege adding, 'He had no doubt been involved in many other incidents where he was able to resolve or control a situation.

It is a tragedy that this situation unfolded and resulted in his death.'

However, there were many lessons to be learnt from this tragic event, most of which could have been prevented the unfortunate outcome. The court heard that the officers at the scene failed to factor in the mental illnesses of Fiona Barbieri and her son, who had been calling out obscenities to the police and emailing rants to politicians during the siege.

They failed also to factor in the weapons that may have been in the house, the aggressive big dogs or accessing the COPS records that would have helped them to assess the risks involved dealing with the pair.

Further, the critical incident investigation team found that an initial plan to distract Fiona Barbieri to one end of the house while attempting a forced entry at the other end, was somewhat flawed. Mainly because there were too many variables: the house was dark, the weapons unknown, the dogs would most likely attack them and they would know the police were coming (there was no element of surprise). The CIIT found that time was with the police and a policy of 'contain and negotiate' should have prevailed.

The court also heard evidence from Assistant Commissioner Anthony Crandell, Commander of the NSWPF Education and Training Command, that over the last six years, the force had put in place major changes affecting risk assessment and siege response that meant officers were to have significant training on 'high risk' incidents with an emphasis on 'safety first'. Essentially, specialist officers were more focused on gaining evidence than producing a safe environment. In addition, he gave evidence as to the establishment of a 'Lessons Learnt Unit' that sought to address the systemic police issues in a timely manner.

Near the end of the inquest, Mrs Donna Anderson was heard to say of her extraordinary husband, 'I have never harboured any doubt that, with his final breath, the welfare of his staff would've been at the forefront of his mind.'

A fitting tribute to a true hero.

Epilogue:

In the three years after the Barbieris were arrested, the Commonwealth Bank foreclosed on the 5-acre property and on 8 June 2013 the property went up for auction. Keven Waters bought it for $830,000. The Barbieris' initial fear that Mr Water wanted to buy their property at a 'rock bottom' price became a self-fulfilling prophecy.

The Barbieri bastion, a former fortress of fear, was subsequently demolished.

The Wife Over the Cliff Killer: The Desmond Campbell Case

This is a rather sad case where a lonely, loving, honest and trusting country woman was duped into marrying a man who was more interested in getting access to her money and two properties inherited from her late husband, rather than giving her the love, care and attention she very much deserved.

★

Desmond Campbell has been described as a liar, swindler, womaniser, gold-digger and now, a cold-hearted killer who pushed his wife off a cliff. To add a further twist to the story, he used to be a police detective with the Victoria Police for nine years. He left the force in 1994 after having been handed a suspended two-month jail term for assault, along with a series of disciplinary matters that were looming.

Janet Fisicaro, 49, met Desmond Campbell in 2003 when he was working as a paramedic in Deniliquin in southern New South Wales, where Janet had lived most of her life with her family. Campbell had managed to seduce a number of women before her and get them to marry him. Janet was to be his third wife.

When Janet first met Des Campbell she was a widow who had lost her husband Frank Fisicaro, some six years earlier. But Des Campbell had a sordid secret past.

Long before he met Janet Fisicaro, he was a disgraced Victorian drug squad officer who used violence to get confessions out of suspects and apparently planted false evidence to incriminate them. In 1994 he left the force 'under a cloud' and moved back to Britain, his country of birth, where he joined the British police in 1995. But while working as a constable in Surrey, he began dating a woman by the name of June Ingham, a married traffic warden. She accused him of indecent assault and the allegations were forwarded to the Crown Prosecution Service, but initially no action was taken.

He subsequently left Britain for Australia due to the implementation of a police internal disciplinary enquiry. He clearly realised they were onto his case and decided it was time to leave.

Eventually, Campbell found work within the NSW Ambulance Service where he met up with Janet Fisicaro. He was working as an ambulance officer and living beyond his means, so was regularly in debt. A romance developed after he met Janet at Deniliquin Hospital, where Janet worked as an orderly. Using a combination of charm and deceit, he won her heart. She was besotted with Campbell.

Janet had now developed a serious relationship with a truly 'bad boy'. Unfortunately, she decided to marry Des Campbell, much against her family's approval. They didn't like him and many efforts were taken to talk her out of marrying him. They were worried that he was just after her money.

How right they were.

However, Janet, 49, still went ahead and married Desmond, 52 in secret on 17 September 2004 at a charming country inn by a marriage celebrant.

She was a lovely bride. She wore a cream-coloured suit and had her hair done for the occasion. She carried a sheath of orchids and appeared very happy. However, the glow disappeared when the conversation turned to her absent family members. Curiously, no-one took any photographs of the wedding.

The celebrant, Jennifer Whelan, later commented that the newlyweds didn't seem to spend a lot of time together and in her view, they appeared to be a 'mismatch'. It wasn't the usual joyful wedding.

The following month Janet purchased a house in Otford, a suburb north of Wollongong, near the Royal National Park, putting it in both their names. Janet stayed living in Deniliquin for six months after they married and only moved to the Otford property on 18 March 2005.

In the meantime, Campbell had moved straight into the house along with three other girlfriends that stayed with him from time to time. All this occurred without Janet's knowledge!

Janet moved back from Deniliquin to Otford in March 2005 after telling her family that she had married Desmond Campbell. It had been a tough call for her.

Six days after she moved in, Campbell arranged a camping trip to the nearby Royal National Park. Janet was a novice camper and was afraid of heights. Clearly, Campbell did not consider either of these concerns of his wife, as he pitched their tent just metres from a 50-metre cliff drop.

Here was a man with a plan – and as it turned out, an evil plan.

It was a warm evening of 24 March 2005 as the couple settled down in their camping site. After a nice evening meal it was time for bed. But first, it was time to visit the 'loo'. Being in the bush, there were limited facilities so she headed to what she thought was a private spot. Little is known what happened next, but it appears her husband followed her and carried out the deadly deed.

Her dead, broken body was subsequently found at the bottom of the cliff.

Campbell used a rope to climb down a nearby gully and found her body on rocks at the base of the cliff. Flattened vegetation along with a telling footprint and several broken tree branches on the clifftop showed Janet had made a desperate attempt to save herself. To no avail. It was a tragic ending.

Campbell rang 000, telling the operator what he believed had happened. A police rescue team arrived, along with detectives and crime scene officers who examined the area, taking photographs of the scene and Janet Fisicaro's body in its final resting place.

The rescue officers and forensic experts then abseiled down the cliff to examine Janet's body, which was winched up from the base of the cliff and taken to the local hospital for death certification and then onto the Glebe Mortuary.

What investigators found was that the tent was pitched close enough to the cliff edge for Janet to have gone over accidentally – but also so close police were suspicious and suspected foul play.

A subsequent week-long inquest was held into Janet's death before the Deputy State Coroner, Jacqueline Milledge, a former police prosecutor, whom I'd previously given evidence before in the earlier inquest into the tragic death of Dianne Brimble. Much of the earlier information surrounding the fatal incident was brought up as evidence during the enquiry.

However, unlike Ms Brimble's case, no drugs were detected in Janet's body. Not even a sedative drug such as diazepam or alcohol, which may have eased the terror of her last days of life.

It soon became apparent that throughout Deniliquin, Des Campbell had a reputation for being a womaniser and was considered something of a 'rogue'. In contrast, Janet Fisicaro was a homely, naive and devoted country lady. Yet, his courtship of the unsuspecting Janet was kept so quiet that few were able to warn the wealthy widow as to what he was up to.

There were many other revelations to follow, including those from three former girlfriends who described him as a persuasive and manipulative and while still maintaining the appearance of a charming man.

One thing that didn't go unnoticed at the inquest, was how physically similar Campbell's victims were. They were all attractive blondes in their middle years, who were either widowed, divorced or just plain lonely. His perfect victims.

The first evidence came from a former girlfriend, a British woman by the name of June Ingham, whom he revealed to that he had nothing to his name but an old Falcon car. But he begged her to come to Australia after her divorce in 2000. However, when the divorce settlement was much less than Campbell expected, Ms Ingham was dumped at the airport. But, amazingly, he later convinced her to buy a house and put it in his name. What was she thinking?

True to form, he sold the house while she was overseas and then broke up with her via a text message.

The second former girlfriend of Campbell to give evidence was Linda Rodgers. She told how Campbell spent a fortune on fine food and expensive French champagne to seduce her at an exclusive Melbourne hotel only a few months before he married Janet Fisicaro.

Then, he followed up with explicit emails to Linda Rodgers, a month after Janet had died, asking whether she would go on an overseas holiday with him.

It was all very inappropriate.

Linda told the court, 'He'd been wooing me and he was married to someone else. He should have been a grieving widower.'

She then broke down in tears, saying to the court, 'It's very humiliating. I'm very embarrassed. I'm very sorry. I'm very sorry to the family. It's terrible.'

Throughout the inquest, the witnesses in general, maintained their composure and even sense of humour, despite the difficult circumstances. One instance, said it all.

When June Ingham (one of Campbell's earlier girlfriends) told the court that he spent a great deal of time on the computer. She was asked by Patrick Saidi, SC, counsel assisting the coroner, 'What was he doing on the computer?'

June replied with an embarrassed smile, 'He said it was banking.'

Ms Milledge then quipped, turning to the court reporter, 'That's banking with an "A".'

That comment, broke the tense atmosphere, bringing a moment of comic relief to the courtroom.

Strike Force Saltwater was subsequently formed to investigate the incident and detectives further delved into Campbell's background. What they found wasn't pretty.

He was confirmed to be a well-known womaniser, swindler and 'gold-digger'. But, to top it off, he used to be a police officer and had spent nine years with the Victoria Police Force. He subsequently left the force in 1994 with a series of disciplinary matters pending and having just been given a suspended two-month jail term for assault.

Much of this information confirmed earlier reports. But like they say in the television advertisements, '… but wait, there's more'.

Campbell supposedly declared to a Melbourne newspaper that there was wide-scale corruption within the police service, and that it was, '… one endless roller-coaster of lies, fabrication of evidence, perjury, stealing and scams.' He went on to say, 'I was just scum. I became like the people I was arresting.'

Maybe so, but he was unrepentant and still carried on with the corruption.

But the matter didn't end after Janet's fatal clifftop fall.

Campbell decided not to attend his wife's funeral, and after being widowed for a week, sought a copy of Janet's will. The previously besotted and now deceased lady, had changed her will to leave him almost half of her estate with the balance to her son.

Campbell then turned his attentions to one of his earlier girlfriends, Gorica Velicanski, taking her on a holiday to Townsville. And like his previous lovers, Ms Velicanski did not know he was married. Nevertheless, he proposed to the woman, who wisely turned him down.

And Janet Fisicaro was in her grave only some four days earlier!

Undeterred, Campbell turned to the internet and landed a further victim in the Philippines, a month after Janet's funeral. Her name is Melissa. She was to become Campbell's fourth victim.

But, sadly there were to be further victims in the form of two children she had with Campbell, now of preschool age.

By now, the prosecution had enough evidence to convict Desmond Campbell.

It was a pleasant, though partly cloudy, sunny Tuesday morning when the Desmond Campbell's murder trial commenced on 13 April 2010, before Justice Megan Latham in the NSW Supreme Court in Sydney.

The Crown Prosecutor, Mark Tedeschi, QC, started by alleging that Desmond Campbell, 52, had carefully chosen the site to dispatch his 49-year-old wife Janet saying, '… that it was a most unlikely, uncomfortable and unsafe camping spot that one could imagine.'

Mr Desmond Campbell had previously pleaded not guilty to murder.

Mr Tedeschi stated that, 'The Crown case is that the accused's relationship with Janet Campbell, from beginning to end, was motivated by how much money he could get from her. He merely saw her as a source of large amounts of money. His marriage to her was a complete and utter sham.'

Crown Prosecutor Mark Tedeschi told the court that Mr Campbell's motive for killing his wife '… was sheer greed for money.'

The court further learned that in the weeks leading up to his marriage to Janet Fisicaro, Campbell was seeing other women and even maintained relationships with three of them after his marriage.

Mr Sean Hughes, SC, appearing for Desmond Campbell, admitted that his client might justifiably be regarded as '… a philanderer, a womaniser, a cad and perhaps even a gold digger. But not necessarily a murderer'.

He urged the jury not to be influenced by what they thought about the accused man, and reminded them that he had pleaded not guilty to murder.

Further evidence was provided by various forensic police officers and by Professor Rod Cross, who formed the opinion from the witness box that Mrs Janet Campbell was most likely pushed off the cliff.

Then, in May 2010, before sending the jury out to consider their verdict, Justice Latham advised them not to be swayed by sympathy for Janet Campbell nor by the immoral activities of her new husband that had been heard as evidence. However, the judge concluded that Des Campbell's attitude towards women could 'inspire revulsion'.

Not surprisingly, the jury returned a guilty verdict.

Campbell stood stony faced as the verdict was read out.

Justice Latham sentenced him to a non-parole period of 24 years expiring on 9 May 2034 with a balance of nine years expiring on 9 May 2043.

Then, in early 2014, Des Campbell's legal team appealed against the conviction on four grounds, which included the 'prejudicial' evidence provided by retired physics professor Rod Cross. This was remarkably similar to the appeal launched by Gordon Wood, Professor Cross having given evidence in both cases relating to the physics of cliff falls. Ms April Francis, Campbell's barrister, told the NSW Court of Appeal consisting of three judges, Chief Justice Tom Bathurst, Justice Peter Hidden and Justice Carolyn Simpson, that Professor Cross's expertise was not relevant to the fall involved, as Mrs Campbell's shoe print was found at the scene. She added, he wasn't an independent witness as he was engaged by the Crown.

The judges agreed that it had not been properly determined that Professor Cross had 'the relevant expertise, derived from both study and experience, to provide the expert opinions that he did.' However, they were 'satisfied beyond reasonable doubt of Mr Campbell's guilt on the evidence properly admitted at trial' and dismissed the other three grounds of the appeal.

The earlier sentence stood, with Campbell's earliest release from prison dated at May 2034.

Curiously, if Des Campbell had shown some affection for his wife he may have got away with murder. But then, if it was genuine affection, he would not have carried out the foul deed anyway. Further, suspicions may not have been aroused if Campbell had turned up at his wife's funeral or waited more than a few days before seeking out the contents of her will. In addition, he may have been seen as a grieving widower had he not taken one of his several lovers on a luxurious holiday the week Janet died.

But Janet was besotted by Des Campbell and would not listen to her worried family; she was sure that she would be with Des Campbell for the rest of her life.

Sadly, she had no idea how little of that life she was to enjoy.

An Incident at a Nursing Home: Murder by Insulin

'Be careful who you trust,
the devil was once an angel.'
– Anon

Ballina is a delightful seaside town on the far north coast of New South Wales. Located 737 kilometres north of Sydney via the Pacific Highway, it's only 90 kilometres from the Queensland border. With eight superb beaches, it's a haven for surfers and tourists alike.

But Ballina isn't just all about beaches, because this scenic seaside town also plays host to a number of quality aged nursing homes, including the St Andrew's Village aged-care facility, in which this story unfolds. St Andrew's is a privately operated nursing home with 117 residents (at the time of writing), and it offers care levels ranging from low-care hostel-type accommodation to high-care nursing home facilities. Residents occupy their own rooms and are cared for by nursing and care staff. The facility operates round the clock, seven days a week, and has staff to cover each of the three daily shifts - morning, afternoon and night.

★

Eighty-two-year-old Marie Darragh, 77-year-old Isabella Spencer and 88-year-old Marjorie 'Madhi' Patterson were residents of the St Andrew's Village high-care nursing facilities known as the Dianella 1 and Dianella 2 wings. Marie Darragh and Isabella Spencer were in Dianella 1 wing, while Marjorie Patterson was in the adjoining Dianella 2 wing. Apart from Isabella, who had type 2 diabetes, all three residents just had the usual medical ailments associated with old age, such as cardiac conditions, arthritis and other associated problems.

On the evening of Friday 9 May 2014, Megan Haines (previously known as Megan Dickson), a registered nurse (RN) and divorced single mother of two dependent children, Ashely Haines, aged 12, and Zack Chalmers, aged four, began her night shift at St Andrew's Village at about 10 pm. On duty with her was a care service employee (CSE), Marlene Ridgeway, who had been at the facility for a number of years and had been working the night shift in the Dianella wing for about 12 months. Three other CSE staff were also in the facility in various other areas, although being the RN, Megan Haines was the one in charge and therefore the one who was responsible for the administration of medication to patients on that shift.

At about 11 pm that evening, the Director of Care, Wendy Turner, visited St Andrew's Village and met with Megan Haines, handing her written notification that complaints had been made against her. Furthermore, she was informed that the complaints had been lodged by Marie Darragh and Marjorie Patterson. Arrangements were made for a further meeting to be held the following Tuesday. It looked like Megan Haines' job could be on the line.

Wendy Turner left the facility around 11.40 pm and Megan Haines returned to her RN duties in the Dianella wing, no doubt seething from the news. But duty called. Just after midnight, Marlene Ridgeway left Megan Haines alone in the Dianella wing, as she was required in another part of the nursing home to assist other staff, returning after about an hour so they could begin their joint round. Before they started, they visited Marie Darragh's room, where they heard groaning noises. They listened for a while with Megan Haines commenting, 'Oh, she's just having a dream.'

The two of them then went on to minister to the various residents, with Megan Haines seeing to Isabella Spencer, and Marlene Ridgeway seeing to a neighbouring resident.

After completing the round at about 2.20 am, Megan Haines told Marlene Ridgeway about the two complaints against her and talked about how it may affect her nursing registration. They then went to the nurses' station, where they attended to general administration duties and answered resident call button requests as needed.

Before beginning the second round of the night, they signed out Schedule 8 medication for a resident. During the round, Megan Haines indicated that Isabella Spencer was fine. However, no checks were made on Marie Darragh or Marjorie Patterson. The round was completed at about 6 am when their shift concluded, and they handed over to the day staff, which comprised an RN and her CSEs, who later found both Marie Darragh and Isabella Spencer sweating heavily in an unconscious state.

The RN promptly contacted Dr Jerome Mellor, the on-call doctor, for advice. He prescribed pain care and advised that both patients be transferred to Ballina Hospital, saying that he'd come to oversee the transfer and make examinations of the two women. However, before the transfer could be made, both Marie Darragh and Isabella Spencer passed away in the presence of their families and friends.

Meanwhile, Marjorie Patterson complained to Dr Mellor and the St Andrew's Village staff that she'd been woken during the night by Megan Haines and given unscheduled pain medications, so she was transferred to Ballina Hospital for further observation and blood tests.

Due to the circumstances and the unexpected deaths of Marie Darragh and Isabella Spencer, death certificates were not issued and the matter was referred to the police for further investigation.

Later the same day, it was determined that an open ampoule of Mixtard 30/70 insulin, prescribed for resident Edward Capewell (a diabetes sufferer), was missing from the medication room in the Dianella wing. Subsequently, police set up and secured crime scene areas in the rooms where Marie Darragh and Isabella Spencer had been residents and in the Dianella wing medication rooms. Crime scene examinations were carried out after a warrant had been granted by Parramatta Local Court. On completion of those examinations, the bodies of both Marie Darragh and Isabella Spencer were transferred to Lismore Base Hospital morgue.

On 11 May, prior to their transfer to the Department of Forensic Medicine in Newcastle for post-mortems, several sets of blood samples were taken from the two deceased women to be analysed for insulin and C-peptide concentrations. The post-mortems were completed by Dr Vuletic on 13 May, but he was unable to establish a cause of death for either of the women. Additionally, no natural causes of death could be established. Further blood samples were taken

A blood sample taken from Marie Darragh at post-mortem (at Lismore) was found to have present frusemide less than 1 milligram per litre, morphine (free) 0.03 milligrams per litre, morphine-3-glucuronide 0.05 milligrams per litre, paracetamol less than 5 milligrams per litre and temazepam 0.02 milligrams per litre. Likewise, a blood sample (at Newcastle) taken from the same woman at post-mortem was found to have present morphine (free) 0.02 milligrams per litre, morphine-3-glucuronide 0.06 milligrams per litre, paracetamol less than 5 milligrams per litre and temazepam 0.02 milligrams per litre.

Frusemide (also known as furosemide) is a sulphonamide-type drug which is used as a diuretic and antihypertensive. It's available under the trade name Lasix and is used in the treatment of oedema and fluid retention.

Morphine is an opiate analgesic for the treatment of moderate to severe pain. The usual dosage of morphine to treat pain in adults is between 5 and 20 milligrams, given by injection every four hours, if needed. However, an individual with heightened reflex excitability of their nervous system may take two to three times the ordinary dose and suffer few, if any, side effects. For example, a patient with severe pain from renal colic or coronary disease may be given 45–60 milligrams of morphine before pain relief is obtained and their respiration won't be seriously affected.

Generally, the toxic dose of morphine for a non-addicted person is somewhere in the region of 60 milligrams, and serious symptoms are usually experienced after doses of 100 milligrams. A therapeutic dose of morphine ranging from 5 to 20 milligrams (average 10 milligrams) in a 70-kilogram adult produces a blood morphine concentration of 0.04 to 0.10 milligrams per litre, whereas, 55–65 milligrams of morphine taken intravenously can result in a blood morphine concentration ranging between 0.8 to 2.6 milligrams per litre, leading to profound respiratory depression. The therapeutic range for morphine is given as 0.05–0.12 mg/L. Marie Darragh's blood morphine (free) level was 0.03 mg/L and morphine-3-glucuronide 0.05 mg/L, which indicated she'd received a therapeutic dosage for pain relief.

Paracetamol (acetaminophen) is an analgesic (pain relief) and antipyretic (fever lowering) drug used in the symptomatic management of moderate to mild pain and fever associated with illnesses such as colds and influenza. It's often combined with other drugs, especially codeine, to provide stronger pain relief. The usual adult dose, administered orally, is between 500 and 1000 milligrams every four to six hours, up to a maximum of 4 grams (4000 milligrams) daily. The blood concentration of paracetamol was less than the therapeutic range (10–20 mg/L) and indicated that the drug had been ingested sometime earlier.

Temazepam is a benzodiazepine-type sedative which is available under several trade names, including Normison, and it's used for short-term management of insomnia in adults. The blood concentration of temazepam was less than the therapeutic range (0.3–0.9 mg/L) and, once again, indicated that the drug had been taken sometime earlier.

The blood sample taken from Isabella Spencer at ante-mortem was found to have present gliclazide less than 1 milligram per litre, temazepam 0.05 milligrams per litre, oxazepam 0.005 milligrams per litre, sertraline 0.14 milligrams per litre and paracetamol less than 5 milligrams per litre.

A further sample taken at post-mortem was found to have present gliclazide less than 1 milligram per litre, temazepam 0.06 milligrams per litre, oxazepam less than 0.005 milligrams per litre, sertraline 0.08 milligrams per litre and paracetamol less than 5 milligrams per litre.

Gliclazide is a sulfonylurea derivative, which in turn is an oral hypoglycaemic drug. It's available under various trade names such as

Glygard, Glyzide, Glucomed, Nordialex and Diamicron, and is used for the treatment of non-insulin dependent diabetes mellitus where the blood sugar (glucose) is higher than normal. The therapeutic blood concentration of gliclazide was 0.7–4.9 mg/L, which indicated the drug had been ingested sometime earlier.

Oxazepam is a pharmacologically active metabolite of temazepam, as well as a drug in its own right. The blood concentration of temazepam was less than the therapeutic range (0.3–0.9 mg/L) and indicated that the drug had also been taken sometime earlier.

Sertraline is a selective serotonin re-uptake inhibitor (SSRI) anti-depressant which can result in dizziness and drowsiness, and so care should be taken with any activity that requires alertness and judgement, particularly early in treatment. It's available under the trade name Zoloft and is used to treat anxiety and depression.

The blood concentration of sertraline was within the therapeutic range (0.05–0.25 mg/L) and again indicated the drug had been ingested sometime earlier.

The blood concentration of paracetamol was also less than the therapeutic range (10–20 mg/L), once more an indication that the drug had been taken sometime earlier.

The upshot of all of the above is that the medications administered to Marie Darragh and Isabella Spencer appeared to be consistent with the hospital records and the needs of the respective patients.

However, the endocrinology and glucose results for the two deceased women were inconsistent and provided a different story.

A blood sample taken from Marie Darragh on 11 May was found to have present insulin 134 H mIU/L (milli-international units per litre) [<=9] and C-peptide 0.08 L nmol/L (nanomoles per litre)[0.26–1.73].

A vitreous humour sample taken from her and tested on 12 May was found to have present glucose less than 0.3 mmol/L, while a blood sample taken from her and tested on 16 May was found to have present insulin 2 H mIU/L [<=9] and C-peptide <0.05 L nmol/L [0.26–1.73]. A urine sample tested on 20 June was found to have present glucose less than 0.11 mmol/L.

Essentially, Marie Darragh's blood glucose level was too low.

A blood sample taken from Isabella Spencer on 11 May was found to have present insulin 53 H mIU/L [<=9] and C-peptide 0.05 L nmol/L [0.26–1.73], while a further blood sample taken from her and tested on 20 June was found to have present insulin 1 H mIU/L [<=9] and C-peptide <0.05 L nmol/L [0.26–1.73]. A urine sample tested on the same date was found to have present glucose 0.4 mmol/L.

Insulin is a peptide protein hormone that is produced naturally by the pancreas. It consists of two polypeptide chains with a combined molecular weight of 5808 and regulates the metabolism of carbohydrates and fats in the body by promoting the absorption of glucose from the blood to skeletal muscles. Excess carbohydrates are stored as glycogen, mainly in the liver and muscles, and any carbohydrates that cannot be stored as glycogen are converted by insulin into fats and stored in the adipose (fatty) tissues. Insulin also promotes the uptake of amino acids and their subsequent conversion into protein. It's present in the body at a constant level in order to remove excess glucose from the blood.

When the blood glucose levels fall below a certain level, the body begins to use the stored sugar (in the form of glycogen stored in the liver and muscle) as an energy source through a process known as glycogenolysis. However, when the blood glucose falls too low (into the range of 20–50 milligrams per decilitre (mg/100 ml), symptoms of hypoglycaemic shock develop. They include double or blurry vision, headache, hunger, shaking or trembling and progressive nervous irritability, which lead to fainting, seizures, sweating, shallow breathing, hypotension and coma. Insulin overdosage (insulin shock) causes hypoglycaemia, the treatment of which generally involves the administration of glucose or glucagon.

The initial insulin levels found in the deceased women were as follows:

Marie Darragh

134 H mIU/L (milli-international units per litre), blood sampled on 11 May, the day after her death. A follow-up sample taken on 16 May showed an insulin level of 2 H mIU/L.

Isabella Spencer

53 H mIU/L, blood sampled on 11 May, the day after her death. A follow-up sample taken on 20 June was found to still have present insulin 1 H mIU/L.

Insulin has been used as a means of committing homicide in the past, and given the elevated insulin levels detected in both of the deceased, it was felt prudent to measure the level serum C-peptide in their blood. Serum C-peptide is an inactive remnant of exogenous proinsulin, and it can provide an indication of exogenous insulin administration.

The serum level of C-peptide is normally within the range of 0.7–3.3 ng/ml, and an elevated value for the insulin/C-peptide molar concentration in post-mortem blood does not generally exceed 1.0. It's therefore seen as a useful indicator of exogenous insulin injection. However, the time of testing should take place within 24 to 48 hours of the post-mortem because C-peptide degrades more rapidly than insulin.

The initial C-peptide levels detected in the deceased were:

Marie Darragh

C-peptide 0.08 L nmol/L (nanomoles per litre), blood sampled on 11 May, the day after her death.

Isabella Spencer

C-peptide 0.05 L nmol/L, blood sampled on 11 May, the day after her death.

Marie Darragh was being treated by Dr Chris Greenway for a variety of medical conditions, including cardiac problems, pruritus (itching), arthritis and back pain, but not diabetes (type 1 or 2), while Isabella Spencer was being treated by Dr Colin McDonald for a variety of medical conditions, including right myocardial infarction, left hemiplegia (stroke), urinary incontinence, hypertension, renal calculi, dysphagia and diabetes mellitus type 2.

More importantly, neither patient was an insulin-dependent diabetic.

However, Marie Spencer was taking the oral anti-diabetic drug gliclazide for treatment of her type 2 diabetes.

Following discussions with other experts in the area, I concluded that given the amount of insulin detected in both the deceased's blood, together with the presence of C-peptide/glucose levels in both incidents, it appeared to be consistent with fatal doses of insulin administration.

As events unfolded, I wasn't called to give evidence on that matter, only on whether the other medication given at the nursing home to both of the deceased had been appropriate. After closely inspecting their medical records, I soon realised that the other nursing staff of the Dianella wing had carried out their duties according to the patients' needs and hospital protocol.

The 'fly in the ointment' was Megan Dickson (aka Haines) RN.

In the meantime, the police had been very busy. Strike Force Odimi had been formed to investigate the suspicious deaths, with Odimi standing for versatility, enthusiasm, agility and unconventional methods. I really don't know where they come up with these 'Strike Force' names!

But more importantly, Megan Jean Dickson (aka Haines) RN was subsequently arrested after being extradited from the southern Victorian town with the lovely name of Seaspray, and charged with the aged care home murders.

The matter then went before Justice Peter Garling in the Supreme Court in Sydney on 3 November 2016.

Evidence was presented to show that on 9 May 2014, within a month of Megan Haines starting her new job at the St Andrew's Village aged care facility, three elderly residents had complained about her, and the following morning two of them had been found dead.

The jury also heard some details about Megan Haines' eventful nursing career, which included three prior professional misconduct findings in Victoria. The Crown also alleged that she realised that another complaint investigation could be potentially disastrous for her career, given her past misconduct findings.

Following a two-and-a-half-week trial, it took the jury just a few hours to find her guilty on two counts of murder. She showed no emotion as the verdict was read out.

But more was to follow.

The jury hadn't been made aware of the full details of Haines' chequered history, namely the ins and outs of the previous damning misconduct findings, with alleged drug convictions, assault of patients, theft of jewellery investigations, and previous insulin misuse allegations, which had been picked up following routine blood tests that had detected the presence of elevated insulin levels in two elderly patients at Box Hill Hospital, Melbourne, Victoria, in early 2008.

In addition, jewellery of both patients had gone missing and the only nurse on duty in the ward at that time had been Haines. Police had searched her home in the suburb of Boronia, but failed to find the pieces, so nothing had come of the investigation. No doubt, the jewellery had been pawned off. They had, however, found a small amount of cannabis, and had brought a charge for drug possession.

Sadly, suspicion had fallen on all the nursing staff, until investigations subsequently revealed Haines to be implicated.

In February 2008, Haines had been stripped of her registration by the Nursing Board of Victoria due to misconduct, and when she'd applied to have it reinstated a year later, she'd been refused because a third misconduct investigation had still been in progress.

She'd made another application for her registration in 2012 after legislation had changed the watchdog system from a state to a federal model, and on that occasion, she'd been successful. That, of course, had set in motion the chain of events that had led to the two murders.

Sentencing was set for the NSW Supreme Court on 16 December 2016. Megan Haines sat in the accused box as her sentence was handed down. She alternated between looking up at Justice Peter Garling and down at the floor, never making eye contact with the family members of the victims.

Justice Garling stated Megan Haines' actions amounted to '… conduct almost too awful to contemplate and cannot be tolerated.' Adding, 'Her conduct was deliberate and calculating. It was a gross breach of trust and flagrant abuse of her power. She clearly abused that position of trust. I consider this to be a significant aggravating factor.'

The then 49-year-old Megan Haines was given a maximum sentence of 36 years in jail, with a minimum of 27 years. She will be eligible for parole in 2041. By then, she will be almost as old as her youngest victim, Isabella Spencer.

Rodney Spencer, Isabella's brother, was so overcome with emotion that he had to leave the court. On departing, he said, 'I knew I'd lose a sister sooner or later, but not in those circumstances, and listening to what the judge said, it started to get to me,' as tears started to well up in his eyes. But he was very pleased with the sentence Megan Haines received.

The chief executive of St Andrew's aged care facility said that the former nurse's sentence acknowledged the pain and suffering that had been endured by the family and friends of the victims.

Could these tragic events that unfolded have been prevented? Most possibly.

Ms Haines received a second chance to sort out her life before it again impacted on the elderly. She had a tarnished background before being appointed to the nursing staff at St Andrew's Village aged care facility, Ballina.

So, who was responsible for the appointment of the dubious nurse? The Medical Board? The nurse's registration board? Or the Health Care Complaints Commission?

In reality, probably all of them. With better communication, the true nature of the nurse's dubious background would have been known and appropriate preventative action could have been taken.

Were lessons learned from this case?

Hopefully, yes, for all professionals concerned and for the better treatment of any future elderly patients that may come under the 'care' of less than caring medical professionals.

How Megan Haines will fare during her term in prison is anyone's guess, as prison inmates generally consider it to be 'a dog act' to kill old ladies.

I can't disagree.

Acknowledgements

I would like to thank my former colleagues at the Clinical Forensic Medicine Unit:

Drs Anthony (Tony) Moynham (Director), July Perl, Susan Jennings and Stuart Anderson. Along with the many police officers (both New South Wales and Australian Federal Police) and folk at the Department of Public Prosecution I had the privilege to work with and to discuss the many case matters we had to deal with as a team.

In particular, I wish to thank Detective Sergeant Barry Fay (retired) and his former colleague, Detective Superintendent Ron Stephenson (sadly deceased) who inspired me to write many of these stories.

I wish also to acknowledge Charles Miranda of *The Daily Telegraph* who 'fine-tuned' my story on the Bogle–Chandler case and even included much welcomed archival material.

Thank you to my wonderful family and close friends, whose encouragement helped make this book possible.

My thanks to my publisher, Lesley Pagett, for her skills and understanding, it was a pleasure working with you. To the wonderful team at New Holland Publishers, thank you for your efforts.

About the Author

Sitting Bull, (c. 1831-1890) a famous Native American Indian Sioux chief once said *'Do not let the poisons of the world pull you from your path.'* Curiously, the opposite was true for Dr William J. Allender. His path has led him to many poisons (and drug) cases and the need to help various authorities to prosecute the villains who chose to use them in their nefarious and evil deeds.

As a forensic toxicologist, Dr Allender (or 'Dr Bill') has been called to give expert witness evidence in a number of very high profile cases involving drug overdoses and poisons (including pesticides), in which those substances have been used in suicides and murder. He has also given evidence in coronial matters that have become so emotional that the court has had to be adjourned for members of the family to compose themselves.

As for the many other cases, a number stand out due to the unusual or macabre circumstances: one involving the mysterious deaths of a brilliant scientist and a nurse by a riverside (Misty River Mystery: The Bogle-Chandler Case); the horrific murder of a man by his butcher lover (The Aberdeen Butcher: The Horrific Crimes of Katherine Knight); a young woman found murdered in a shallow bush grave with a dead dog for a 'pillow' (A Dog and a Dame in a Ditch: Who Murdered Maureen McLaughlin?); a morphine poisoning of an aged veteran by his supposed carer (The Black Widow: A 'Morphine Mistress'), just to name a few.

First published in 2021 by New Holland Publishers
Sydney • Auckland

Level 1, 178 Fox Valley Road, Wahroonga, NSW 2076, Australia
5/39 Woodside Ave, Northcote, Auckland 0627, New Zealand

newhollandpublishers.com

A record of this book is held at the National Library of Australia.

ISBN 9781760794101

Group Managing Director: Fiona Schultz
Publisher: Lesley Pagett
Project Editor: Liz Hardy
Designer: Andrew Davies
Production Director: Arlene Gippert

10 9 8 7 6 5 4 3 2 1

Keep up with New Holland Publishers:
NewHollandPublishers
@newhollandpublishers